W9-AJM-407

Praise for

A BREAST CANCER ALPHABET

"*A Breast Cancer Alphabet* is a brisk, user-friendly ABC of dealing with the disaster of cancer and how to get through it with a smile. It is a remarkably insightful and sensitive guide to making the best of the worst, all delivered with Madhulika's wit and vital energy." —**Tina Brown, former editor of** *Vanity Fair,* *The New Yorker,* **and the** *Daily Beast*

"Madhulika Sikka's *A Breast Cancer Alphabet* is brilliantly researched, smart, and personal—an unvarnished primer of what every woman needs to know about the diagnosis, treatment, and consequences of living with breast cancer. Her practical advice from A to Z is exactly what I wish I'd known when I was first diagnosed. With the trained eye and ear of a top-flight journalist, she demystifies the disease, telling you everything you forgot to ask that no one else will share. Reading it will help you recognize, and even laugh, at your worst fears. B is for Brava, Madhulika, for your honesty and creativity in guiding us on a journey none of us chose to take. It is a lot easier when you have *A Breast Cancer Alphabet* at your side." —**Andrea Mitchell, NBC News chief foreign affairs correspondent**

"Breast cancer is a topic no woman wants to learn about first-hand. But should it happen to you, Madhulika Sikka's *A Breast Cancer Alphabet* is an ideal primer for before, during, and after the experience. Offering the kind of real-world advice that can only come from someone who's lived to tell the tale, Sikka's book is required reading for anyone in search of a book that will bring you up to speed quickly, gently, and with genuine empathy." —**Micki Myers, author of** *It's Probably Nothing . . .*

A BREAST CANCER ALPHABET

CROWN PUBLISHERS · NEW YORK

A Breast Cancer Alphabet

Madhulika Sikka

All rights reserved.
Published in the United States by Crown Publishers,
an imprint of the Crown Publishing Group,
a division of Random House LLC, a Penguin Random House
Company, New York.
www.crownpublishing.com

CROWN and the Crown colophon are registered
trademarks of Random House LLC.

Library of Congress Cataloging-in-Publication Data
Sikka, Madhulika.
    A breast cancer alphabet / Madhulika Sikka.—First
edition.
    1. Breast—Cancer—Miscellanea. I. Title.

RC280.B8S4963 2014
616.99'449—dc23   2013003652

ISBN 978-0-385-34851-5
Ebook ISBN 978-0-385-34852-2

Printed in the United States of America

Book design by Elizabeth Rendfleisch
Illustrations and cover design by Roberto de Vicq de Cumptich

10   9   8   7   6   5   4   3   2   1

First Edition

For Sushma

&

Krishan Lall Sikka:

It all begins with Mom and Dad

CONTENTS

A BREAST CANCER ALPHABET

INTRODUCTION

There is a hushed reverence in the waiting area outside the Oval Office. After all those years of *The West Wing,* one might think there would be a bustle of activity—a swirl of smart, earnest people walking and talking at the same time. Perhaps I would catch snippets of conversation about budgets and bills, policies and politicians. It's not like that. My NPR colleagues and I were there to interview President Obama, and we waited quietly with a stenographer and the Secret Service. No one else came by.

Despite my years of journalism in Washington, it would be my first time in the Oval Office. It was December 2010, and the White House was beautifully decked out for the holidays. It should have been an exciting moment, but the only thing I could concentrate on was my cell phone. Four days earlier I had undergone a needle biopsy on a suspicious mass in my left breast, found after a routine mammogram. I was waiting for my internist to call with the results. In my heart I knew it would not be good. Something in the radiologist's manner gave me a clue. As she prepared for the biopsy, I'd tried to break the ice.

"Maybe it's just a blocked duct," I'd said jokingly. She didn't laugh or even crack a smile. Not good, I thought.

This was also the week when Elizabeth Edwards died after having been diagnosed with breast cancer just six years prior. The wife of the onetime presidential and vice presidential candidate John Edwards, she had revealed her diagnosis a day after the 2004 presidential election, in which her husband and his presidential running mate, John Kerry, lost. Her cancer returned in 2007 during her husband's bid for the presidency. She ultimately weathered the twin challenges of breast cancer and her husband's infidelity with grace and poise. I had pored over all the reporting about her in the days since my biopsy. Of course this was part of my job as a journalist, but it took on greater meaning for me as I awaited the results of my biopsy. Thoughts of her passing went through my mind as I paced nervously and made small talk with my colleagues.

On a nearby table, there was a digital photo frame

cycling through images of the president. For some reason I kept waiting for the photo of then Russian president Dmitry Medvedev and President Obama at Ray's Hell Burger, the renowned hamburger joint in nearby Arlington, Virginia, to come round. Why was I so taken with that picture? Maybe it was because I had eaten there myself with my husband and two daughters, and I remembered how we'd laughed at the contrivance in this photo, the presidents of two superpowers, in shirtsleeves, just enjoying a burger like any old Joe. I felt my phone buzz and saw the caller ID was blocked. I didn't answer. This was not a conversation I could have. Not here, not now, waiting to be called into the Oval Office at any moment.

All I remember about my entrance into the Oval Office was that the room seemed much smaller than in the movies. The Christmas tree was also surprisingly understated in its decorations. Was the furniture more shabby chic than stately home? Couldn't tell you. The new rug? No idea. I can tell you that the president looked older than I had imagined. Twenty minutes after we had entered the Oval Office, we were done. Extending the Bush tax cuts, the

START treaty, overhauling the tax code—the topics raised in the conversation whizzed by in a blur. The president stepped out to the outer office and donned his coat and scarf before heading off to light the national Christmas tree. We gathered our equipment and headed to the NPR filing booth, a tiny closet located underneath the press briefing room (formerly a swimming pool), to file a quick clip of the interview with the president for the top-of-the-hour newscast. I ducked out of our booth to check my voice mail. One thing to know about the filing area under the press briefing room is that cell reception is quite bad. I had to wander around to find the place where my phone would actually work. Anxious and pessimistic, I listened and breathed a sigh of relief. The call was from my middle school daughter's teacher, apprising me of something that had happened at school that day. Normally I might have been concerned about a call from school, but given what I was anticipating, this was welcome and not worrying news.

I returned to the filing booth, where we plotted out what we would be doing for the next news cycle, what clip we could play later in the evening, and the next morning's show. My job as executive producer of *Morning Edition*, NPR's flagship show, which reaches some 6 million listeners a day, was all about decisions—big and small. How would we use the president's interview with host Steve Inskeep throughout the broadcast? Was there a role for our White House correspondent, Scott Horsley? What clip would we put out in advance of the morning's broadcast and release to the press?

I left my colleagues Steve and Scott to structure an outline for our story and wandered back upstairs to the press briefing room. You know this room, the one that has the blue curtains with the White House logo and the press secretary's podium. It is the site of the daily press briefing. Here you get a cell signal. I noticed a fresh voice mail. It was my doctor asking me to have her paged.

The moment of reckoning had arrived. I needed some privacy for this conversation, so I stepped outside, into the crisp, cold early-evening air as I waited for the hospital operator to track her down. There was a construction site right by the briefing room, a massive hole with big pipes sticking out. It might as well have swallowed me up. My head had been full of the president's interview, and now my doctor was delivering the most devastating news I had ever had in my life: "You have breast cancer."

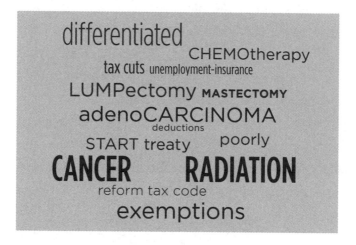

What my doctor was saying competed with words from the president's interview in this word cloud in my head. I was shaken back to earth when she added, "Here is the first thing you are going to do. I've made you an appointment with a breast surgeon, and I will get one for an oncologist."

There was a plan. The producer in me appreciated that my doctor knew that there needed to be an action item to go with the delivery of this news. But it was Thursday night, and I wouldn't see the surgeon until Tuesday. No decisions would be made on my cancer for some days. Nothing to do for now except go back to the office at NPR headquarters and make decisions about things I did have some control over: how to edit the president's interview for air the next morning, how to divide the interview between the two hours of the show, how to work with our digital team to have it all ready to publish online, and how to craft a press release with our communications department. And of course, I had to decide which pizzas to order while we were working on all of this. Five hours after getting the diagnosis, with the interview in good shape for air, I crawled into a taxi and went home. My husband, Jim, had been out that evening performing at a holiday party with his band, a hobby he pursued with vigor outside his duties as a Georgetown University history professor. I hadn't called him because I knew he would be onstage and would probably not even hear the call. As it happened, we both got home around the same time. The kids were already asleep. We didn't have to say anything to each other. He knew as the tears welled up in my eyes. I curled up on the couch with him and cried.

I'm in the information business, so my first instinct could have been to get on the Internet to see what I could find out. But I knew that doing this would send me down the rabbit hole of unbridled fear. My husband had been diagnosed with cancer a decade earlier, a rather rare tumor in his salivary gland, and just a short time on the Web looking up information about his condition had convinced me that he was going to die soon and I would be left a widow before the age of forty with two young children. He didn't and I wasn't. In fact we had just passed the ten-year mark since his diagnosis, and his health today is excellent.

In the days between diagnosis and the first surgeon's appointment, the mind makes mischief. There is nothing to do but wait and overthink. The lump in my left breast had grown from the size of a pea to the size of a clementine—in my head. I would not survive to see my kids graduate from high school—in my head. I would never visit my dream city, Istanbul—in my head. What was I supposed to do to keep myself distracted?

I needed a filter for the volume of information that was out there. Fortunately, my brilliant friends Anne Gudenkauf and Alison Richards, both of whom are science journalists, became my cancer coaches, preparing me as well as we prepared for an interview with the president. I gathered both of them in Alison's office and sat down.

"It appears that I have breast cancer, and I really need your help to get me ready to meet the breast surgeon," I said. At this point all I knew was that the biopsy showed a "poorly differentiated carcinoma." What did that mean?

"It means you have cancer," they told me. "They like to check the other breast more closely, so you'll probably have to have an MRI," Alison said.

"But I'm really claustrophobic," I said. She could sense my anxiety but gently insisted that it was a good thing for me to do.

My friend Anne is one of the wisest and calmest people I know. "We'll put some things together," she said. "There are some helpful websites that spell out the questions." They came up with key questions that I needed to take in to the doctor with me. What kind of breast cancer do I have? Has the cancer spread? Will I need surgery? What kind—lumpectomy or mastectomy? What tests do I need to have before the surgery? Who is going to be my doctor and coordinate my care? I was fortunate to have a prep team who understood the science of oncology and who weren't as emotionally racked as I was. My longtime friend and colleague Cokie Roberts, who herself had been diagnosed with breast cancer almost a decade earlier, was also an enormous help in those early days. When she asked how my family had reacted to the news, I told her that only Jim knew and that I would tell my girls, my father, and my siblings after that first appointment with the surgeon. I wanted to wait until I had a plan before talking with them.

"You are not going to walk out of that office on Tuesday with a plan," she warned me. "That's going to take a while."

Cokie proceeded to tell me the questions I should ask that would give me a sense of the steps I would be taking over the next few weeks. Would they look at the sentinel nodes during surgery? If they did, I'd be staying overnight, so I should plan to have someone with the kids while my husband was with me. Would I know the characteristics of the tumor right at surgery time? Would I be going in for a lumpectomy? If they found something else, would they do more invasive surgery at the same time? And by the way, she was right about not having a plan after that first appointment!

Cancer treatment is a whirlwind. As one friend said, "This cancer stuff keeps you busy!" I reverted to my journalistic instincts, asking questions, seeking guidance, being persistent without being too pushy. Soon it became clear that I was heading for a single mastectomy, and it was likely I would also need chemotherapy, though the pathology on the cancer could not be done until the tumors (yes, plural) had been removed and had gone through extensive analysis.

I was also inundated with literature, from the American Cancer Society, from the Lombardi Cancer Center at Georgetown University, where I was being treated, from the nutritionist, the social workers, and my friends. I had a big box full of information about mastectomies and chemotherapy and nutrition and drugs. The great thing about living in the twenty-first century is our access to information. Unfortunately, the bad thing was that I was being drowned by information—so much of it and with so little time or head space to look at it clearly and objectively.

But none of this information really helped me: me the woman; me the mother; me the wife. *Me.* Nothing prepared me for the emotional loss of my hair or for the fact that my breasts would become the domain of *so many* people and would even be photographed, regularly. Nothing clued me in to the fact that I would be so exhausted I would flop on my couch like a rag doll. Nor did any of the official literature make me aware that a few strategically placed pillows would dramatically ease my discomfort during post-op recovery. I didn't then know that I would discover extraordinary acts of kindness in every facet of my life, or that I would be able to laugh about my plight sometimes.

Women with breast cancer are expected to be upbeat, but also hard-assed and martial in their attitude about the disease. We are constantly told that we can beat the cancer, but when you are actually going through the treatment, you often feel helpless as the true effects of it take hold. I thought, If I didn't have any say in getting the disease, why would I be able to beat it? No one told me it was okay to cry uncontrollably or okay to be angry or okay to acknowledge out loud that it is a real bummer to be diagnosed with cancer.

I needed something that would validate how I was feeling at particular moments. A little pick-me-up that I could turn to—nothing too long or scientific or self-indulgent, something that I could slip into my handbag or have by my bedside that I could dip in and out of. A short book that wouldn't tax my chemo-addled brain. Something that filled the gaps in the overflow of information available at the touch of a keyboard, something that spoke to me the patient. Where would I find that? Sadly, breast cancer has become an epidemic, with 250,000 new diagnoses every year in the United States alone. One in eight women in the United States will be diagnosed with breast cancer. With those kinds of odds, it was not surprising that I had many friends and colleagues who were fellow travelers in Cancerland. They were my guides, who helped me navigate this treacherous terrain. But not everyone can rely on friends like mine who happen to be science writers or media professionals.

So this is a book for anyone who has been diagnosed with breast cancer and needs a companion. This book is for all of you who have become members of a club you did not want to join. This book is for your friends and relatives who are going through this with you and may not always know exactly what you are feeling. Above all, I hope that this book will sometimes put a smile on your face but *always* let you know that you have every right to feel the way you do on any given day. It sucks to get cancer.

"A" IS FOR ANXIETY

Here's the truth: the anxiety starts really early, well before you are even diagnosed. It starts when you get the follow-up letter after a routine mammogram. Before that moment you've never given your "routine" mammogram another thought. *It was recommended that additional mammographic views and possible breast ultrasound be performed.* The letter doesn't seem to be too anxious, but you certainly are. Then your anxiety ratchets up when you go back to the clinic and while you wait for the doctor who is looking at your mammogram. When she doesn't crack a joke with you but rather looks so earnest and concerned about a mass that isn't a shadow but an actual mass, the jig is up. Anxiety is often triggered by the anticipation of future events, and all you can anticipate are bad things.

You have to make an appointment for a biopsy. This is the first thing you need to do, before you see a surgeon, before you see an oncologist. The biopsy will identify what the thing inside you is. Until the doctors know exactly what they are dealing with, they are no good to you. Why can't I do the biopsy now? Because there are orders and papers and signatures and schedules that are not in sync with you and your anxiety. So you hurry up and wait. While hours and days pass, the anxiety has run rampant. A mass that you might not have even felt before is now giant; you don't even have to press hard to feel it, and every time you do feel it, it seems to get bigger. Then there is the interminable wait after the biopsy to see if what you have actually is breast cancer. While you wait, your future life rushes before your eyes, a life you think you will not be part of: your kids' high school graduations, weddings, births, travel to places you'd always wanted to visit.

Once you are diagnosed, the inevitability of treatment as well as the unknowability of treatment stoke the anxiety that darkens your door. In my case, it was a mastectomy followed by chemotherapy. As you await the day of surgery, a sly glance down at your chest allows you to imagine what the new geography of your body is going to look like, and as you wrap your head around the notion of breast removal (see "M Is for Mastectomy"), this imagining is anxiety inducing. Anxiety grips you as you await the pathology results in the days after they remove the breast and study the tumor. When you know you have to have chemotherapy, you try to anticipate what your body will feel like after it has been pumped full of poisons to cure you. Because there is nothing to prepare you for all of this, your anxiety meter will be off the charts.

Anxiety is different from concern, even from worry or fear. You can be worried about the state of the world or concerned about the ozone layer or scared of dogs or bees. Anxiety is something altogether different. Fear is something all animals experience, but anxiety is unique to humans. It is also part of living with cancer. It doesn't define living with cancer. Anxiety is more like your cancer companion; it is attached to you now, sometimes in the background, sometimes front and center, but always there.

From the prosaic to the profound, I always found a reason to be anxious. Will I get a bed or a recliner at the chemo infusion unit? Are they giving me the right drugs in the right dosage? Are they sure I don't need a prophylactic mastectomy? Anxiety stalks you as you sit through countless doctor visits, hours and hours of tests, and days and days of waiting. Anxiety actually sinks its tentacles in you and makes itself at home through bad news and even when you get some good news. It lurks like an unwelcome visitor who never leaves, because it never does. Anxiety is in your mind, yes, but it also manifests itself physically— nausea, light-headedness, stomach upset, racing heartbeat.

Your challenge is to manage it. I'm pretty good at time management and, if I put my mind to it, weight management too. Anxiety management is a completely different beast. Anxiety is not neat or measurable. It is amorphous and stubborn and oh so resilient. It cannot be compartmentalized or shoved aside or thrown out or vanquished. It actually must be managed, and you have to figure out the best anxiety management techniques for you. It can be drugs (see "D Is for Drugs"); it can be therapy of a wide variety of types (see "T Is for Therapy"); it can be meditation or yoga or work or play or ice cream or movies. Coping with anxiety is the part of your cancer treatment that may get short shrift from the medical professionals. They are dealing with a big thing—your cancer—and thank goodness for that.

But anxiety is real and important, and you have to let people know that so you can get all the help you need to manage it.

So why doesn't it go away? Maybe you've gone through all the prescribed treatment and your doctors feel good about your prognosis. So how come the anxiety is still there? Because once you have cancer, all you can think about is, Will it come back? Every ache and pain you have that might be a result of aging or strenuous activity or an accident, they all could be your cancer coming back. At least that is what you think and that is what you get anxious about.

The good news is that reality is never as dark as the places your mind can take you, and unfortunately anxiety takes you to the darkest places imaginable. Maybe living with it becomes a learned skill and the anxiety subsides; in the meantime, managing it seems to be the only option.

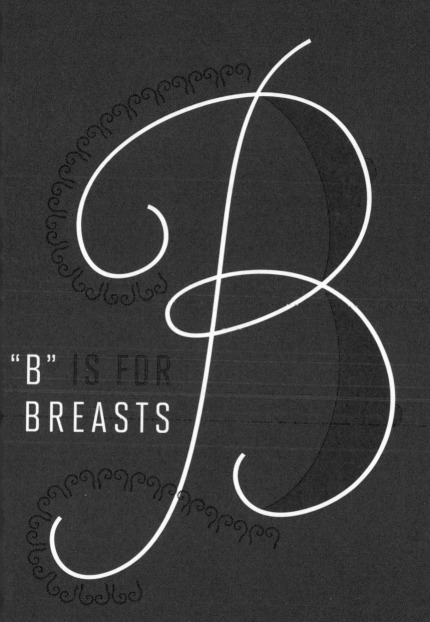

"B" IS FOR
BREASTS

Breasts. Bosom. Bust. Knockers. Tits. Rack. There are so many ways to describe the protrusions on your chest that you are unconsciously aware of the moment you see your first Barbie doll. Mammary glands start developing in your teens and become the focus of much angst as they grow. Regardless of their size, their mere being seems to dominate your physical presence in a way that no other part of your anatomy can. Breasts are what make you sexy, voluptuous, a woman, perhaps a mother. Breasts are so fetishized in the public discourse that it is a surprise when you think about it that they are pretty private for most people.

Have you ever photographed your naked breasts? Have you ever had someone else photograph them? I suspect the answer to both those questions is no. When did you ever talk about your breasts in public? Probably never or not very much. But then suddenly, with this diagnosis, it is *all* about your breasts. As soon as you are diagnosed with breast cancer, you start to feel the stares of people, even if they *aren't* staring at you. You think people *are* taking a furtive glance down at your boobs as they are talking to you, because really that *is* what you are talking about. Suddenly the plastic surgeon is snapping away, taking photographs of your breasts "before" so he knows what to do "after."

Since when did talking about your breasts become okay? Well, when you have breast cancer it becomes sort of okay. If you were having your leg amputated, or part of your colon removed, you wouldn't really have any problem discussing that. It's because of the highly sexualized nature of the world we live in that our attitude to breasts is different. "They are cutting off my boob" is what you want to say, but you don't. We have this sterile-sounding medical term—*mastectomy*, which is now part of everyday parlance. I, however, see it as an amputation of the breast. All of a sudden you find yourself engaging in matter-of-fact conversation with your brother, your male colleagues, maybe even your neighbors about a part of your body you never, ever would have discussed before.

I have sat in a waiting room where women of all ages are talking about their breasts! Across the room so all can hear. "I love my new breasts," says one.

"He does such a good job," says another. Friends who have gone through what you are about to go through offer to show you their breasts! I actually touched the breasts of one friend to feel how much softer and more natural the silicone implants feel after a temporary expander, which feels like an alien interloper in your chest (see "R Is for Reconstruction"). Doing so made me feel so much better about what I was about to go through. That friend's offer was a wonderful gesture. Friends promise to go bra shopping with you when you are "all done" and have become the owner of a fabulous new silhouette. "You are going to get the rack of a twenty-four-year-old; it will be fabulous," my dear friend David told me. Who knew? The bright side of a seemingly terrible diagnosis.

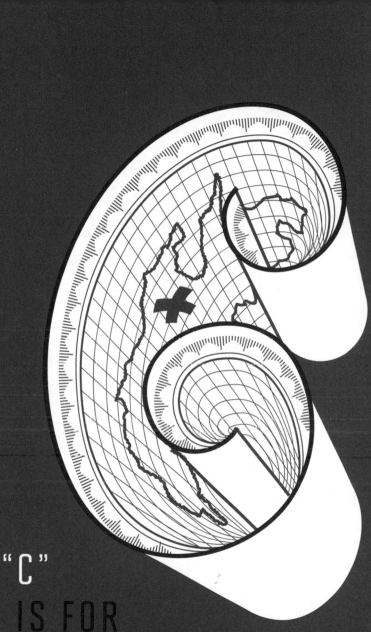

"C"
IS FOR
CANCERLAND

I have been fortunate enough to travel a lot. In fact, my husband and I have been to some amazing places around the world, and there are some places we've wanted to revisit but haven't got to yet.

However, there was one place that we had no intention of ever going back to. In 2000 my husband was diagnosed with cancer and we entered Cancerland. He went through successful treatment and we became visitors emeriti, always somehow associated with Cancerland but only around the edges. Sadly, in 2010 I was diagnosed with breast cancer and we were back, both feet firmly planted in Cancerland.

I'm one of those anal types who like to plan for a trip. Maybe it is the broadcast producer in me. Before going to a new place, I make folders full of travel articles, restaurant reviews, notes on hidden gems to visit that I'd find out about from friends and acquaintances. I also like to have some sense of a schedule: to know where I'm landing, where I'm staying, what to see, and how long my trip is going to be. Well, here's the thing about Cancerland—one minute you are minding your own business, living your humdrum life, and the next minute you are thrust into this strange land of surgeries, and drugs and side effects, and pain and anxiety, and you didn't even have a minute to prepare for it.

It's like stumbling through the wardrobe into another world—you are about to embark on a mysterious trip and you don't know where it is going to end. You've received no notice, no clear map, and no schedule.

Usually when you plan a trip for yourself you have a sense of who your fellow travelers might be. When you are backpacking in the mountains, there will be the healthy, active types. Exotic locales not much visited yet will have intrepid, adventurous types. You know what I mean. You feel you can identify with at least some of your traveling companions.

The thing about your fellow travelers in Cancerland is that they can be anyone. Cancer offers absolutely no barrier to entry: young, old, rich, poor, male, female, white, black, athletic, sedentary. Cancerland is not the slightest bit discerning about whom it will allow to visit. The only criteria—some rogue cells running around your body. That is your passport, visa, and ticket.

There are some things worth knowing about Cancerland. The first thing is that it is an incredibly busy place, and you will be astounded by how many people are there. The place where you get the best sense of that is the chemotherapy infusion unit. Being there is like going to a public beach on the hottest day of the year. Patients spewed out of the waiting room into the corridors whenever I arrived there. And even though I had an appointment, there was the wait, always the wait, because demand so far exceeded supply; it's a little like being double-booked except you're waiting for the next free recliner or bed so that your daylong session of poison pumping can start. At all my visits to the chemotherapy infusion unit, it was standing room only. I half expected to hear an announcement like at a train station: "Please stand clear of the doors, another train is following shortly."

But there are some stops in Cancerland where you *are* treated like those people who can boast of fast-track access, where you don't have to wait with the hoi polloi but instead just get ushered in ahead of everyone else. When you are undergoing treatment you get your blood tested, *a lot*. Not for me the long wait in the main lab at the hospital full of people with *other* ailments. There was a secret lab, just for those of us in Cancerland. In and out in fifteen minutes, every week.

I hope you will not have to go to the emergency room during your treatment. I, sadly, did. When you are really sick, the idea of an endless wait to be seen makes you feel worse. Well, not in Cancerland. I found myself being wheeled in immediately. "Make way, chemo patient coming through." Small comforts, I know, but hey, you take what you can get.

Here's another thing to know about Cancerland: the people who are your trip planners—the doctors—have more than likely not visited themselves. They are experts, of course, and they have packed off so many people to Cancerland that they talk a good game, almost like they know what it's really like. They are full of knowledge and tips, things they've learned from visitors who report back. But they haven't actually experienced it the way you and their other patients will. The nurses are more like hotel concierges. They'll tell you what to expect on your visit and what to look out for and what to avoid, but they have probably not been there themselves either. Even the most experienced of the health-care professionals don't know what it is like to feel as tired as you will (see "X Is for eXhaustion") during chemotherapy or how bloated you will feel on steroids, or the extent to which a mastectomy really hurts.

This is precisely why it is worth seeking out the counsel of others who *have* been to Cancerland, so that they can share some of their experiences with you. You will find it is like entering a secret society. You might have known someone who has had breast cancer treatment, and you might have thought that you sort of understood what she was going through. But it is not until you yourself are diagnosed that you realize there was so much you could not possibly know from the outside. Only when you are in the club yourself are the full details of what to expect shared. What your friends share will not be a complete map to Cancerland, because everyone's map is unique, but it gives you the broad contours of this place that once you enter you never really leave.

"D" IS FOR DRUGS

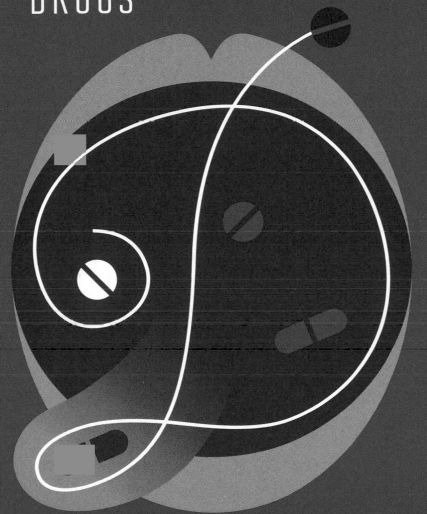

Drugs are your friends. Let me repeat, drugs, pharmaceuticals of all kinds for all things, are your friends. Pill-popping, vein-coursing drugs are your friends. I'm not talking mother's little helper pills from the 1950s, nor do I want to come across as a caricature from *Valley of the Dolls*. I never experimented with drugs in college. I drink organic milk, cook meals from scratch virtually every day, don't smoke, barely drink, and have few processed foods in my house. But I am down with the drugs that have helped me since this ordeal began. I'm talking about the benefits of the advancement of science, ladies.

In the category of silver linings, the fact that you are a breast cancer patient in the twenty-first century counts as one. Trust me. BC (before cancer) I always considered myself healthy. An annual visit to the doctor and ibuprofen for the unyielding onset of middle age, but that was pretty much it for me. Apart from the occasional bacterial stomach ulcer, I've been fortunate not to need a vast array of drugs for anything. Then came my diagnosis, and my dresser became a veritable drugstore.

Here's a peek into my medicine cabinet during the first year of my breast cancer treatment:

Cyclophosphamide, docetaxel, dexamethasone sodium phosphate, famotidine, diphenhydramine, ondansetron hydrochloride, Neulasta, Emend, prochlorperazine MAL, alprazolam, zolpidem, citalopram, diazepam, tamoxifen, hydrocodone, cefadroxil, clonazepam.

There are probably others, but you get the idea.

Lest you be concerned, I'm down to just a couple now. But this list and then some were my companions during the worst part of my treatment.

Many of us think of breast cancer as a modern disease, but it has been with us since recorded history began. Ancient Egyptians, the Greeks, and the Romans all diagnosed and tried to treat breast cancer. Unlike many other cancers, breast cancer was a disease that had an identifiable manifestation—lumps that were palpable, visible, that sometimes even broke through the skin. It is no surprise that from the earliest days cutting was the pretty standard way to treat breast cancer, from removal of the breast with a knife to the more professional early-twentieth-century radical mastectomy with anesthetics. This was, for the most part, a solution to what was considered a local disease, not a disease caused by cellular disruption that required holistic treatment.

I speak as someone who has undergone a mastectomy, so why the faith in drugs? Because mastectomy alone isn't always enough. In the absence of a cure, survival rates are what we must cling to, and clearly chemotherapy, that toxic cocktail of poison that is pumped through our bodies, must count as one of the blessings of late-twentieth-century medicine.

As much as I hated going through it, I tried to imagine chemotherapy as a nail-biting race. The mastectomy had cleared away the lead vehicles, the tumors, which had lodged themselves in my breast ducts, but there was a real possibility that some cells might be running around my body trying to build new tumors. They may have gotten a head start, but now my team had the engines revved up, and as soon as the chemotherapy left the starter gate, a mad pursuit was under way, chasing those microscopic cancer cells and eliminating them before they could make their way fully around the course. Boom! Thwack!

Bam! All routes—ovaries, uterus, lungs, bones—No Entry! My hope is that one day we will look back on chemotherapy the way we now look back at bloodletting and leeches: *They poisoned your whole body just to kill some errant cells?* But in the meantime, I, for one, am grateful for it.

Chemotherapy is but one of your pharmaceutical friends. There are many other drugs you become acquainted with during this process. Anesthetics, of course (imagine having your breast chopped off with nothing but a swig of alcohol and a bit between your teeth to stem the pain), and everything else that they give you to go with the chemo, drugs for stemming side effects and preventing nausea; drugs for anxiety and sleeping; drugs for trying to keep the cancer at bay after the mastectomy and the chemotherapy.

Now some of these drugs will make you feel awful, some will make you feel better, and others will help take the edge off. You have to work with your doctor to get it just right for you. But you have to be stoic about so many other things, you don't need to get all holier than thou about the drugs. Who knew?

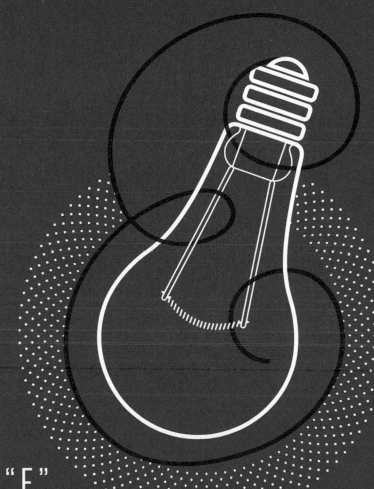

"E"

IS FOR

EPIPHANY

I'd like to say I had one. I'm tempted to say everything in my life changed and I have become a better person. I'd like to say that I unleashed a newfound sense of purpose, a motivation to do all those things I hadn't had the guts to do before. I'd like to say that my cancer has been the most profound thing in my life. Well, it has been, and it hasn't. Don't be too upset if lots of things just stay the same.

Pretty soon after diagnosis you find that the world doesn't stop for you to get off. Your house still gets dirty, the bills still need paying, the roof doesn't stop leaking, your children still need parenting, your parents still need taking care of, and your life goes on in all those quotidian ways it did before. It requires a particular kind of strength to hold your old life together when you have the best excuse in the world to let it all go. I am an ordinary woman, mother, and wife, diagnosed with breast cancer. I am not a Lifetime movie. The lens looking at my life is not soft focus now; if anything it is in sharper relief. The picture is crisp and clear, which is proof enough that life has kept going on.

There are small "realizations," as I like to call

them, rather than epiphanies. You will find that your normally self-centered teenagers have an inner steeliness that shows itself at just the right moment. You will discover that if your husband can't muddle through quite as well as you do, you have to let it go. You will find that the fierceness and loyalties of the women around you are even stronger than you thought they could possibly be. You will discover that even though you are pushing fifty you are still your dad's little baby and his inability to have stopped this disease from entering you crushes him and you love him even more for that. You will find that a part of you is glad your mother is not alive to see you go through this because, as much as you want her there, you know it would crush her too. You will realize your good fortune to be living in the twenty-first century with a disease that millions of people are familiar with and are working to understand more.

You will probably discover that you don't want to pack up and go trek around the world, or build an orphanage for poor girls in Nepal, even if you could. What you want most is your pre-cancer life, which was pretty okay, all things considered, and you would do anything to go back to it. That's what makes you brave and strong and fearless, and it's what most of us have to deal with. I guess maybe that is the epiphany.

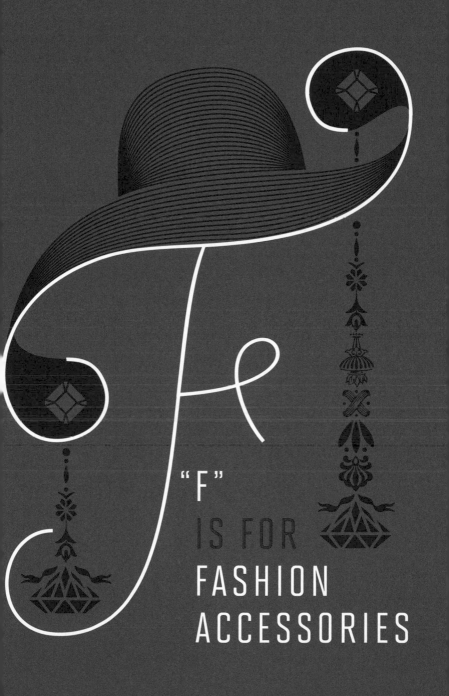

"F"
IS FOR
FASHION
ACCESSORIES

You have been diagnosed with a terrible disease that for previous generations was almost always a death sentence, so it may seem a little frivolous to devote a whole section to fashion, most especially fashion accessories. But frankly, not enough attention is paid to fashion accessories at the best of times, and this is a moment when they come in useful (see "L Is for Looks").

If you undergo chemotherapy, you will soon come to terms with the fact that you are bald (see "H Is for Hair"). Then you will spend an inordinate amount of time figuring out how to cover your head up.

My friend Lesley calls herself a "nostalgist." In her book *Let's Bring Back* she pines for the style and panache of times gone by. Things like handwritten thank-you notes, rolltop desks, and tennis whites. You won't be surprised to hear that she has a lot of time for head coverings of all sorts—hats, head scarves, and turbans; boaters, berets, and safari hats. The world she evokes harkens back to a time of elegance and élan. Here was a bright side. I could use this opportunity to become as stylish and perhaps as divine as many of the heroines of yesteryear.

Chemo headwear is big business. My chemo started in the dead of winter and continued into the summer, so I got to go through some seasons during my treatment. I had a lot of knitted caps courtesy of the hospital volunteers and even my own knitting. I actually needed them, especially at night, because my head would get cold. I didn't expect that. But most of the time I looked like a lumberjack (maybe it had something to do with the open-front plaid shirts I was wearing post-mastectomy) or a cat burglar!

So is there an elegant option? Turbans seemed to me to be the way to go. Elizabeth Taylor died while I was undergoing treatment. She, of course, had a brain tumor removed years ago, and her obituaries were an opportunity to remind us all how gorgeous she looked bald with painted eyebrows during her treatment. Try as I might, I knew I wasn't going to look like Liz Taylor. However, look online and you'll find pictures of her looking stunning in a turban during the 1960s. Sophia Loren and Lena Horne too— carrying off their turbans with grace and glamour. Go back further and find all those brass-balled dames of the 1930s—Bette Davis, Joan Crawford, Rosalind

Russell—they could carry off the turban look without seeming injured or sick or just plain ridiculous. Check out some fashion magazines from the period, and you'll find you can't think of anything more ladylike and chic than a turban on your head (preferably with a large jewel smack in the middle of the front folds) and a fox fur around your neck. Unfortunately, plain ridiculous was how it looked on me. I don't know what it was, maybe you needed a long neck, a larger forehead, or maybe you just needed to see yourself in black and white. "Mom, you look like a chemo patient" was the resounding opinion of my teenage daughters when I tried to go with the ready-made turban look.

Don't worry if the turban is not for you. You will not lack for inspiration—flapper caps, floppy hats, peasant scarves, baseball hats, cloches, straw boaters, and, of course, a wig.

Scarves were my next option. I learned a few things about scarves. Silk slips off your head, so avoid silk scarves if you don't want to spend the whole time touching your head to make sure your baldness is not peeking through. Scarves that are too big and have too much fabric will bunch at the nape of your neck if that is where you have the knot, and they will slip off too. Bandanna-size scarves in thin cotton seemed to work for me, tied in the back not the front (unless you are going after the Rosie the Riveter look). Here is another mystery about the whole covering-up-the-baldness thing. I had black hair. Never colored it, just stuck with my black hair regardless of what I was wearing. Suddenly it became imperative that my head scarves coordinate with my clothes. I had to get a peach-colored scarf to go with my spring clothes, navy for overcast days, gray to look more businesslike, flowery to look more relaxed. Why was I compelled to do this? Was it really necessary that I be all matchy-matchy from head to toe?

There was a time in America when hats weren't just for church. Hats were literally the crowning glory. Bonnets to wide brims, pillboxes to cloches, a lady always wore a hat. I wasn't doing so well with the hats, so scarves were for me.

But if you can't figure out the right head covering for you, bald may be the way to go (especially when it is hot). I found that what really helped me with the uncovered head were earrings. Big, bold, interesting earrings. When people see you bald for the first time, they are a little taken aback, so earrings give them something to focus on. You have license to go a little wild, *and* you are helping the people around you, giving them something to comment on beyond your naked head. That's my rationale, and I'm sticking to it. Hoops, sparkles, stark, shiny—just have at it. You will feel a whole lot better.

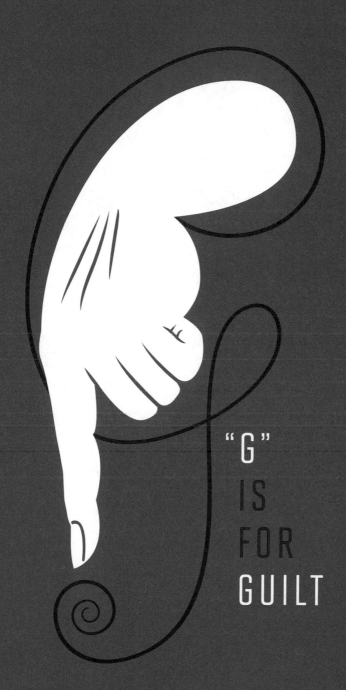

"G"

IS

FOR

GUILT

So, here are some things that might have caused my breast cancer:

Being a woman—guilty
Getting older—guilty
Genetic inheritance—not guilty
Periods before the age of twelve—guilty
Overweight before menopause—guilty
First child after the age of thirty—guilty
Current or recent use of birth control pills—guilty
Large breasts—not guilty
Dense breasts—not guilty
Not breast-feeding—partially guilty (breast-fed for only three months)
Not exercising regularly—guilty
Not having lots of children—guilty
Excessive alcohol use—not guilty

You get the point. You have been diagnosed with a horrible, possibly deadly, disease. You will go through a wretched regimen of treatment and your body will be (temporarily) wrecked as you do. The embodiment of your femininity, the breast, is the treacherous villain in this drama, and *you* are the one who feels guilty. How can this be?

Well, this must have been my fault, right? Looking at that list, I tend to focus on the things that were in my control—weight, birth control pills, breast feeding, exercise, childbearing. Of course I must have done something wrong to cause this, and all I can feel is guilty. With the passage of time you realize this guilt is almost irrational. But that is not what it feels like in the moment. I think that is because not only do you feel guilty that you have this disease you might have been able to prevent (not true, but . . .) but also you start to feel guilty because of what this is doing to the people around you.

You feel guilty that your life at home (which you might have been holding together with duct tape and chewing gum, if truth be told) is going to be severely disrupted by the fact that you have this disease. Your family has to adjust to a new you, a sometimes needy you, a you that isn't really you but a vessel for this disease at this moment.

You feel guilty about how this might disrupt

things for people around you outside your family. For me it was the strain put on my colleagues who were picking up my slack. They couldn't have been more supportive and generous and loving, but that never stopped me from feeling guilty.

You also feel guilty when you hear someone else's story that is worse than yours and so maybe you shouldn't be feeling so bad about what you are going through. And, in case you thought there was nothing that could compound your feelings of guilt, there is. That guilt feels worse because everyone tells you how lucky you are compared with X. There is probably nothing worse than someone who doesn't have cancer telling you how lucky you are. Luck is when you win the lottery (see "O Is for Odds"), not when you get breast cancer.

There is no hierarchy of cancer by which you must abide, where you have to be upbeat and positive because there is someone who has a worse breast cancer than you. That logic might make sense in some detached, objective way, though in fact it is not true. You, the breast cancer patient, are neither detached nor objective. You are intimately attached to this disease, and everything about it is subjective. So, permission granted to feel terrible about what you are going through and to not feel guilty in the slightest about any of it, okay?

Here are the facts about breast cancer. It is an insidious, wretched disease, whose treatment can be worse than the disease itself. You did nothing wrong; you are not being punished for something you might have done in your current life, or your past lives for that matter. The truth is we don't really know what causes breast cancer. Ultimately there is one thing we do know: if you have breast cancer, you have some rogue cells that decided to do their own thing and play havoc with your body. And *that* is nothing to feel guilty about.

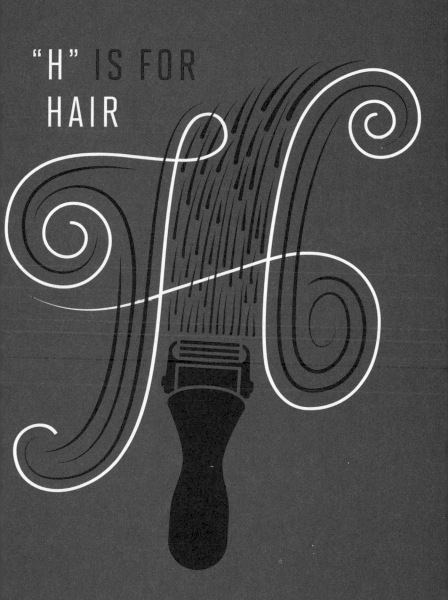

"H" IS FOR HAIR

The term *bad hair day* was invented for women. Hair has occupied an inflated place in our lives since we were little girls, out of all proportion to so much other stuff and certainly out of all proportion to what preoccupies men. (Even sex? *Yes!*) When we were growing up, was hair more important than breasts? I would say yes, though some may argue the two are on a par with each other. How many hours in your life have you spent on your hair—cutting, setting, blow-drying, straightening, curling, crying? Well, to braids, bangs, and barrettes, add bald! If you have chemotherapy, your hair is almost sure to go. Now in the grand scheme of things this may not be such a big deal. Kill the cancer, lose the hair. That doesn't sound like a bad trade-off to the rational mind. But when have we ever been rational about hair? It is okay. You are allowed to be irrational about this one because the hair thing is a *big deal*.

That wretched chemotherapy is a miraculous cocktail of drugs that zeros in on rapidly dividing cells that are growing out of control. But it doesn't distinguish between the bad cells (the cancer) and the good cells—like hair. You have probably thought many times in your life that your hair is out of control. Well, it kind of is. The cells that make up your hair strands are among the fastest-growing cells in your body. You are right: your hair at the cellular level is out of control, and those cells get zapped just like the cancer.

I have tried to imagine myself looking different throughout my life. When I had waist-length hair, I wanted to get rid of it. When it was shoulder length, I had a perm. When it grew out, I wanted to cut it right away. But baldness? That had never entered the equation. You never imagined it either, did you?

So what to do? I have some good news. When you are diagnosed with cancer, you really don't have much control over anything. You think you do, but honestly you don't. However, I discovered one thing I could control. After talking to friends I decided to shave my hair off before it fell out. For some, waking up with clumps of hair on the pillow is a traumatic experience. In addition to the trauma of diagnosis and treatment, you are faced with a hair 911 that must be dealt with right away. I was not going to take that route. There is enough to handle without trying to muscle your way into the salon for an emergency hair appointment.

Here's what you, too, can do: shave it off. I could tell that some around me were a little taken aback. First step? Talk to someone else who has been through this. Get recommendations for hairdressers who have experience dealing with cancer patients. Believe me, they will hold your hand through this process in every way. I had a consult with the wonderful Hans, a gentle soul with the perfect manner who was a Washington institution among women who had gone through what I was going through. I was to discover later that he also volunteered in a program to help women cope with their changed looks during cancer therapy. After that consult, at which I tried on a number of wigs, I made an appointment. Hans encouraged me to bring people along and turn it into a party. So that's what we did. My husband and children, my sister and my girlfriends, sparkling cider and cupcakes in tow, forty-eight hours after my first chemo session I had all my hair shaved off.

I will not deny that the minute he took the razor to my head I was freaking out inside. My teenage daughters looked on bravely, but I knew it was tough for everyone. Don't worry. It moves fast. Your friends are there with you, and before you know it, the hair is gone. Give yourself permission to cry at this precise moment. You've cried for lesser hair misdemeanors, and watching in the mirror as your hair is being shaved off is akin to watching a federal crime being committed. But, I thought, I have a pretty nicely shaped head! This revelation doesn't stop you crying, or your daughters or your sister crying, but it does make you hold your head up a little higher. Make sure you have great earrings on and you are made up. If you have already chosen a wig, have your hairdresser trim it to fit your new bald pate. Voilà! Extreme makeover, cancer style.

Of course I was riddled with doubt. What if I had acted too soon? What if my hair wasn't going to fall out? In fact it didn't, and I was full of righteous indignation. I had stubble that was kind of growing almost immediately after I had shaved my head. "I'm a hard-ass," I told my oncologist. "It hasn't fallen out yet. Maybe I shouldn't have shaved it."

"It will," she said, and she was right. A few days

later my stubble rubbed off on my hands in the shower. The floor looked a little like the sink does after my husband shaves, with tell-tale stubble around. It was still a profound shock, and I cried inconsolably in the shower. But I was grateful I wasn't pulling out clumps of my shoulder-length hair (and clogging up the drain).

Now how about the hair not on your head? That depends on the chemotherapy drugs you are on. Chances are some or all of it will go. Believe it or not, it's not as traumatic as it could be. No eyebrows? Very bad (see "L Is for Looks"). Leg hair? Well, no waxing for the duration of my treatment, so not so bad. The same for underarm hair. For those of us who have inherited the hirsute characteristics of our ancestors, this was some very welcome news.

What happens to your hair is important. There were many times when I was up in the middle of the night and saw a scary thing in the mirror: a bald me with no eyebrows and sallow skin and a face so puffed up from steroids that I looked like a billiard ball or Nosferatu (see "L Is for Looks" again). But I'm here to tell you it passes and your hair grows back really quickly once you have completed your treatment.

In the Hindu faith, there is a tradition to perform a *mundan* on a child's first birthday. The head is completely shaved to rid the child of all the negativity of previous lives, the undesirable traits of previous incarnations, so that the child can start anew. I didn't have one of those when I was one year old, so I approached my haircutting as a *mundan* ceremony forty-seven years delayed—the first step on the road to new, post-cancer beginnings.

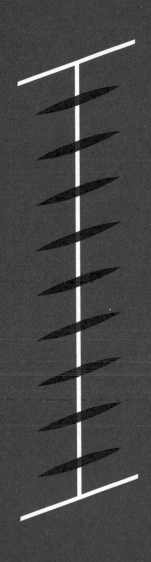

"I" IS FOR INDIGNITIES

If you are aware of the breast cancer culture that has built up in our society over the last two decades, you might think that you are entering a world of fuzzy pink gauze, soft teddy bears, and garlands of ribbons. Generally a land of sparkling brightness personified by women who are happy and smiling while they are "battling" this disease, the "she-roes" (rhymes with *heroes*), as Dr. Gayle Sulik has caustically described them. The writer Barbara Ehrenreich calls this the "bright-siding" of the disease. In this narrative you would be hard-pressed to find stories that were not about triumph over adversity and how breast cancer has made someone a better person. For some, a cocoon of cotton candy somehow cushions this ferocious disease, making it seem nonthreatening, just another part of life's passage, like puberty or marriage or childbirth.

Actually, there is not much in Cancerland that is pink or gauzy, and failing to recognize that is one of the many indignities of breast cancer. There needs to be room to acknowledge some of these indignities, so here is my attempt to do just that.

Even those of us who have not been diagnosed

with breast cancer have, of course, been exposed to the indignity of the mammogram. Plop your breast in between two plates that exert their viselike grip on your boob, hold your breath, take a picture. Take a breath, turn the machine, and do it again. Just a couple of different angles, won't take long.

Then there is the prodding and probing in the biopsy. I wasn't sure how this was supposed to work. A needle biopsy sounded to me as if a needle would be inserted, like a pipette, and a tissue sample would be drawn out from the mass. Actually, it felt and sounded more like a staple gun, inserted multiple times into the lump to remove multiple tissue samples. Try this at home. Staple some paper together using five or six staples, one at a time, and as you do, imagine that happening in your breast. It was the sound that really resonated with me. Ca-chunk. Ca-chunk. Ca-chunk.

For me one of the lasting indignities was the sheer extent to which my breasts were no longer mine. A long succession of people manhandled (and woman-handled!) me. Each professional was perfectly nice and well meaning and above all professional, but they were focused on my breasts, not me, almost as if my breasts were not even part of me but rather just objects in isolation that needed dealing with. Prior to this experience, the people who had an up close and personal relationship with my breasts were my husband, my gynecologist, and my breast-feeding children. Now I was being photographed, perused, and palpated by a rotating cast of doctors, residents, and sundry other medical folks.

X-rays and MRIs—more people who need to work with your breasts. Lie down on your stomach and let your breasts drop into this Plexiglas box. Don't move while we slowly slide your body through this tube.

Oh yeah, I almost forgot about the lymphoscintigraphy. Lie down while we inject this nuclear radiotracer into your nipple and you can watch the dye travel to your lymph nodes right here on this screen. Yes, we do need to do three separate injections into your nipple area. This was a vital procedure, it would help my surgeon as she tried to find out whether my cancer had spread to my lymph nodes, but it did not make those shots in my nipple any easier to endure.

After your mastectomy, drains will be hanging

out of your breast wounds. The drain is called a "grenade drain" because, yes, it looks like a grenade! A tube comes out of your incision and empties fluids and blood into a suction bulb. Okay, I stand corrected, that fluid that comes out of your wound? That's kind of pinkish red, so here is the hint of pink. My drain, which I had in for about two weeks after the surgery, was uncomfortable and annoying. It can flop around if you don't have it in place properly. So you spend a lot of time organizing yourself so that it doesn't catch on something and rip out. Yes, a small thing in the grand scheme of things but . . . still.

And another thing, a nine-inch scar across my chest where my breast used to be (see "R Is for Reconstruction"). Look, my plastic surgeon was really good and did incredibly careful work. But a nine-inch scar is still a nine-inch scar that stares back at you if you look in the mirror, like a gash across the landscape of your womanhood. I knew it was there, I just didn't look for the longest time because my relationship to the way I looked during treatment was complicated to say the least (see "H Is for Hair" and "L Is for Looks" and "M Is for Mastectomy"). And one thing I could not look at was the huge scar across my chest. In fact, I didn't look at it for months and months.

These were my indignities. Yours may be different. My point is breast cancer is many, many things. What it is not is a fun ride. It is painful and debilitating and public, and it is okay to feel indignant about that.

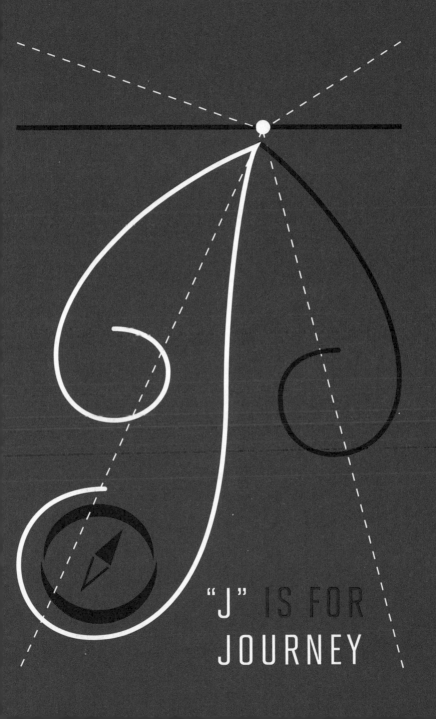

"J" IS FOR
JOURNEY

There is something about cancer that seems to invite folks to liken it to a journey, and not just any journey but a particularly mystical journey. There are so many other diseases that people have to live with, yet no one talks about an AIDS journey, or the journey of heart disease or hepatitis or . . . take your pick. But some people take on that hushed tone of concern when they ask you about your cancer and then you actually tell them about it! They weren't quite expecting that, and they feel they have to say something in response, and for a lot of people that response is "Well, it's all part of the journey."

So I'm going to try to unpack this moniker somewhat—the journey.

In what ways is having breast cancer like a journey? Well, I guess the fact that, once diagnosed, you embark on a path that you had no idea you were heading for might make it seem a bit like a journey, though in this case an unexpected one. Many think cancer has a beginning, middle, and end—diagnosis, treatment, end of treatment—as many journeys do. People are often changed by their journeys, and there seems to be a common consensus that going through cancer should change you. I don't subscribe to that particular idea (see "E Is for Epiphany").

Why does this particular word, *journey,* this noun (which is also used as a verb), irritate me so? Maybe it is because the word *journey* seems so completely and utterly inappropriate and inadequate to discuss a process in which the course of treatment, despite all the advances of modern science, is still slash or poison or burn, or some combination thereof—cut, chemo, radiate, maybe even all three. There is absolutely nothing about enduring breast cancer and its treatment that is like any journey I have ever taken, even the bad ones!

I have been on some remarkable journeys in my life. The first is one I was not even aware of. I was a mere four months old when my parents set sail on a ship from India to England. Another extraordinary journey was the one familiar to so many immigrants, the journey I undertook after marrying my American husband and moving here to the United States.

After a year in this country, my husband and I moved back east from California. We drove along the southern route. I got to see the majesty of the Grand Canyon, the beauty of Zion National Park in Utah, the endless, stark emptiness of Texas, a state that seemed to go on forever, and the hot and humid Deep South. Now *that* was a journey.

I've traveled the deserts and mountains of northwest China. What an amazing journey, sleeping in a yurt in the soaring Tian Shan mountains, riding horses, and getting caught in a jam of fat-tailed sheep! I've visited so many places around the world, some on the well-trodden path of travelers who came before me, others off the beaten track, but all full of excitement and adventure. Those were all journeys.

To me the word *journey* describes something that is rooted in the physical world, transporting from one place to another. To me a journey implies wonder, exploration, perhaps a particular destination. It sometimes has romantic connotations, a journey to the exotic and enchanting.

My breast cancer was not mystical or enchanting or exotic. My breast cancer was not and is not a journey.

Getting through cancer is no different from getting through some other terrible disease because that is what it is, a disease. It's okay to treat it like one.

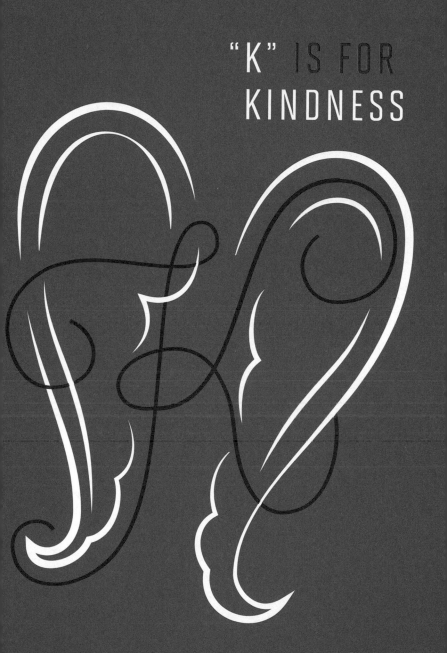

"K" IS FOR
KINDNESS

When you break the news to your friends that you have been diagnosed with cancer, the first thing they will do, after their initial shock and concern, is offer to do something for you. You should think about this. Not too long. Not too hard. Just long enough and hard enough to figure out what you need done and then let them *do it*.

If you are anything like me, you will think that you can handle this, that the systems you have set in place will work just fine and people shouldn't trouble themselves for you. Type A personalities, in particular, take note: you should disabuse yourself of this notion as soon as possible. People really want to help, so make them feel good by letting them and you will feel good too.

You will receive extraordinary acts of kindness and love from people all around you, people in parts of your life whom you might not have given much thought to beyond a perfunctory nod or hello in the morning. You learn to accept this kindness because you like to think that you will be as helpful to them or others should they be in the same predicament. What's more, you actually really need the help, even though you may not know that to begin with.

Sara was one of the kind angels who surrounded me. Using her well-honed instincts as a television producer, she got word out via e-mail to a large list of friends about my diagnosis and treatment. She also used her skills to organize our meals with an online calendar, outlining details of how many to feed and our dietary restrictions. She provided precise delivery instructions and even put a cooler on the porch so we didn't have to answer the door if we weren't in the mood! For five months our family of four was fed by Sara and her battalion of angels, friends, and colleagues from so many spheres of my life.

This single act probably contributed most to preventing the strain that could have disintegrated our family as we dealt with my medical challenge. Our friends all cooked wonderful, healthy, and appetizing meals, and there was one gesture in particular that spoke volumes. Everyone who made a salad made their own dressing! Even after all this time has passed, it is something that strikes me as extraordinary. This seemingly small act spoke volumes about how kind people are and how much thought they put into helping at a time of need.

There is the kind angel who drives you places if

your husband can't be two places at once; the immensely kind angel nurses who stay sunny and upbeat as you are going through the most awful thing in your life; the amazing volunteers at the chemotherapy infusion center—they are very special angels of kindness; the wonderfully kind and loving administrative staff at all my doctors' offices, the frontline troops in your medical mission, handling the vital task of logistics; the parking attendant at the office who parked my car and helped me carry things on the days I did go to work and who made me feel okay about my baldness because under his hat he was bald too. He is an angel, and his name really is Ammanuel. Your friend who had also gone through breast cancer and delivers a wedge pillow that is indispensable (see "P Is for Pillows"); the amazing mothers who take your kids off your hands when you're in need of a break; your self-centered teenage daughters who have enough awareness to know that no matter how much you don't want to, Mom really needs you to hold her hand as she takes a walk around the block just to keep her systems running and alert. Kindness abounds in ways big and small in your life. Embrace it.

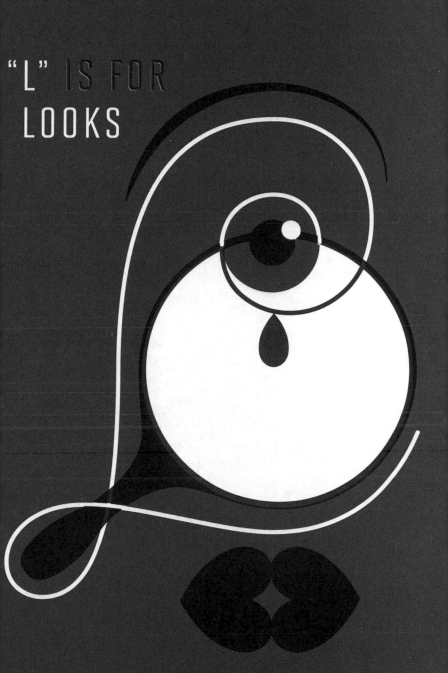

"L" IS FOR
LOOKS

Yes, at this point you might be thinking that some of the topics addressed in this book ("F Is for Fashion Accessories" and "H Is for Hair") are superficial and would be at the bottom of your list of concerns when facing a biggie like breast cancer. Well, there are many surprises that come with a diagnosis of breast cancer, and thinking about your looks turns out to be one of them.

We will stipulate for the record that you are careful about your looks, but not overly concerned. You care in the I'm-a-woman-who-comports-herself-acceptably-to-societal-expectations-and-am-thoroughly-presentable kind of way, not in the I-spend-two-hours-every-morning-primping-and-painting-myself-and-will-not-let-a-soul-see-me-without-makeup-on kind of way. But the thing about breast cancer treatment is that it does things to your looks, and not necessarily good things. So, whichever category you fall into—plain or primped—you find yourself thinking: Why am I so worried about my looks right now? I'm going through breast cancer for goodness' sake. Well, because you are a woman, and it matters more for women. There, I said it. I will spare me my own righteous indignation (and yours) at this point and just accept that this is true (see "H Is for Hair" again).

I am not talking about buying into the whole "crazy sexy" cancer thing here, which is not where my head was, and frankly you can get through cancer without embracing that extreme. As my friend the humorist and fellow cancer traveler, the late David Rakoff, told the *New York Times,* "It seems like the oncological chapter of the covert war on women . . . often preached by women against women, which is often just a variant on the pressure on women to not get epidurals during pregnancy and die in labor like in the Victorian age. It sounds like, 'You should go to chemo in sky-high Jimmy Choos!' And if you don't you're a lazy bitch who deserves to die of cancer."

So no, I didn't go to chemo wearing Jimmy Choos and lipstick. However, I found myself introduced to a program called Look Good Feel Better, a collaboration between the American Cancer Society and the cosmetics industry that provides skin care, makeup, and grooming counseling (including wig wearing and tying a head scarf) to women who are going through cancer treatment. At your first session, during which professionals teach you how to make yourself up, you are handed a big free bag of makeup that suits your skin tone, no doubt to help you look good and thus feel better.

I'm actually someone who has never worn much makeup. So I'm not one of those people who ascribes her cancer to carcinogen-laced makeup. The last time I wore mascara was probably at my wedding. But I have to say I learned a lot of useful things. Things like the importance of applying sunscreen on my bald head—obvious, you say, but no, not really, if you've never been bald. I learned that my nails, like so much else, would suffer. In fact, they turned a blackish purple color, which was quite disturbing. I learned to apply moisturizer with upward strokes and to contour my cheekbones with a powder blush. In all, I was taught twelve steps to make myself up completely. I never did all twelve, maybe eight or nine on some days.

Why was I doing this at all? I'll tell you why. I looked awful during my treatment. Really, it was not a pretty sight. My face bloated like a balloon from the steroids, the chemotherapy made my skin blotchy, I was so sallow there was a ghostly pall about me. And, of course, I was bald. To be completely frank, I felt like crap.

But did I need to look like crap? Like I said, I was going through breast cancer treatment, so it would have been fine to leave well enough alone. Believe me, most days, when just getting out of bed was an achievement, that is exactly what I did. But there were other days when I did something about it. The days I went into work I put aside an extra twenty to thirty minutes to apply my makeup and fit my wig or head covering just right. It was almost like applying a shield, not letting the wider world know just exactly how sick I was or how badly I was handling the treatment. Not because I was ashamed of it, but because, you know, everybody doesn't need to know all my business all the time. Going through something like cancer treatment is hard, and it shows. Providing myself with a mask (literally) protected me from the awkward gazes of the people around me who couldn't help but notice how awful I looked on the days I didn't don that mask. It probably helped them handle my disease better too. That may seem an odd thing to be concerned about, but I was concerned about it because I didn't want my handling of the disease to be an awkward thing for anybody.

I have had male friends and colleagues who have gone through cancer treatment, and I can assuredly say that everything I've just discussed was not in the slightest bit relevant to them. I have tried to instill in my two teenage daughters the sense that looks aren't everything and form just a small and irrelevant part of *who* a person is. So how hypocritical was I, being so concerned about my looks? Like I said, I could not have put on the "face" every single day, or even have put on the full face ever. But there were days when donning the mask really helped. That's not self-centered or vain or egotistical, that's just what worked for me. If it works for you, great, because you and no one but you gets to decide how you look.

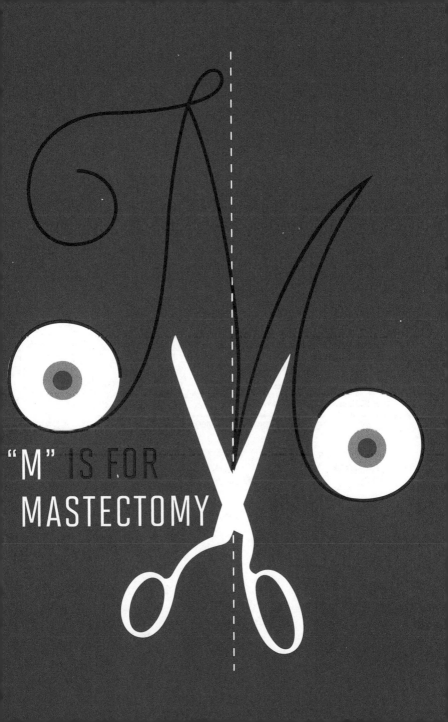

"M" IS FOR
MASTECTOMY

For many women a diagnosis of breast cancer will lead to a mastectomy, sometimes single, sometimes double. Whichever it is, it is an extreme step but, for many, a lifesaver.

The word sounds benign and almost refined, *mas·tec·to·my [ma-stek-tuh-mee], noun, plural -mies. Surgery. The operation of removing the breast or mamma.*

It's a word that is certainly polite enough for company, the subject of open discussion among friends, acquaintances, colleagues with whom you might never have discussed your breasts before (see "B Is for Breasts"). However, if I were to describe this procedure as an amputation of the breast, it would probably make most people recoil. Having been through one myself now, this is how I describe it. Something that was there is now gone, something that protruded from my body is now "lopped" off. The words *amputate* or *amputation* never came up when I was diagnosed with breast cancer. They still don't. The first term used was *partial mastectomy,* commonly known as *lumpectomy.* But soon it was clear that there was more than one tumor and the only course of action was a mastectomy.

Mastectomy is a word that tens of thousands of women hear every year, and it is a course of action they take. It is a brutal, violent thing to have happen to you, and it is perfectly fine to feel that it is an amputation, and don't let anyone tell you otherwise. For me it was easier to cope with by thinking of it in that way. On those truly dark days when you are in real pain, and you look down and the familiar landscape of your body is no longer there, it is a humbling and mournful experience. In my case, one side had been obliterated, in a process akin to mountaintop-removal mining, and there was a flat, stark, scarred space where once had resided a soft, protruding manifestation of my femininity and sexuality. At that moment, *amputation* seems a more accurate description of the procedure than anything else.

At first blush you don't give much thought to what a mastectomy means. *Mastectomy* is a medical term you've heard a hundred times before. In that meeting with the breast surgeon, the overwhelming thought is that there are cancer cells running rampant in your breast and the only course of action is to remove the offending appendage before those little buggers get comfortable and spread throughout your body and claim squatters' rights. Once they make themselves at home, it is always hard to throw squatters out! Get them out of me by any means necessary. It is a visceral reaction. My house has been invaded. Hurry, do it right away. Can we book the operating room soon? How about now? Well, it turned out that we could, relatively quickly, send in the cavalry to throw those invaders out. Ten days after being told that a mastectomy was my only option, I was under the knife, and a few hours later I was down a breast.

I must confess, I've never been much of a boob person. I've always dressed modestly and don't like to show any cleavage. Spaghetti straps were not an option in my wardrobe, let alone strapless. As I got older, I had even less desire to showcase my boobs. Gravity and motherhood certainly took their toll. What miracle of engineering would hold up my breasts without some extravagant superstructure? I wasn't huge, just average, 36C, but always conscious of my not very perky breasts.

So I didn't love my breasts, but they were mine. I wouldn't say I was particularly attached to them or proud of them, but nothing quite prepared me for how awful I would feel when I lost one. There is the physical awfulness, the flattening of your whole body (see "P Is for Pillows"). There is also the bruising and the drains from the wound. Immediately after the surgery you are bound up like an Egyptian mummy, a surgical bra holding you together as drains protrude out of the sides and gunk collects in little containers that you empty every day. You can barely raise your arm, and you need assistance to lift yourself up in bed.

But there is something altogether more dispiriting. This is the worst physical manifestation of the disease. It is there every day to remind you what you have been through. I will admit that I could not look at my naked self in the mirror for months after my mastectomy. I knew I would be having reconstruction, but that was going to be after I was somewhat recovered from my chemo so that I would be strong enough to go through reconstructive surgery. I knew I was misshapen. I knew I had a long horizontal scar across my chest where I used to have a breast. I knew that I would get a new breast, that the doctor would rebuild a nipple and tattoo the areola. I had seen pictures of his previous surgeries. It was actually kind of amazing to see what he could do (see "R Is for Reconstruction"). But I couldn't look at myself. You are covered up, of course; nobody can really tell unless they see you naked. The only people who saw my naked chest were my husband and my doctors. I turned my back to the mirror every time I got out of the shower. In hotels that had walls of mirrors, I never looked up until I had covered myself with a towel.

This may seem like crazy, irrational behavior. In my mind it is the most normal reaction to such a brutal act.

Of course, we are incredibly blessed that in the twenty-first century we are armed with the tools not just to diagnose and remove the cancerous breast but also to reconstruct a breast. For much of the twentieth century the only treatment for breast cancer was what they called a "radical" mastectomy, which also removed the muscles attached to the chest wall. It was a painful and disfiguring treatment. Those were the days before they approached breast cancer as a holistic disease that requires drug treatment as well as surgery. Nowadays, except in the most extreme cases, the muscles are kept in place and it is possible to rebuild your pectoral strength. And of course, you can get a new breast. As my brother reminded me, "You live in America; they have the power to rebuild you." True, but that's a long haul. As you wait to get the perfect boobs, you are allowed to mourn for the lost boobs. A part of your body that defines you as a woman, and maybe a mother, has been removed because it is now host to a disease that could kill you. I can't help but feel that if we called it "an amputation" the rest of the world would get that too.

"N" IS FOR

NOTEBOOK

The day you are diagnosed with breast cancer is a day you will never forget. It is the moment that your world is turned upside down forever. Nothing about you or your life will be the same after that. It is such a defining moment, the moment when you enter Cancerland, you think it is something that you will remember forever. You will now hang on every word uttered to you by every medical professional you will meet. This is a big thing—how can you forget it? Everything about this experience will be etched in your memory forever, maybe even verbatim.

Well, the truth of the matter is, not every word you hear will be carved in stone on tablets that you can pull from the recesses of your memory at will. You will probably remember the diagnosis, I'll give you that. Everything else? That's a little tougher.

As a journalist, I try to bring my inquisitive, analytical outlook to everything I do. I started to take notes from the moment of diagnosis, but it soon became clear that this would not be an easy task for me. There I sat, in the sterile glare of overhead fluorescents, a poster above my head showing a cross-section of the breast and how a ductal carcinoma in situ becomes invasive. My professor husband sat

next to me (also taking notes). I followed along dili-
gently, and then it happened. A tidal wave of fear and
shock washed over me. It was the moment I realized,
Oh, she's talking about me. I lost focus and passed
the notebook to my husband. He continued to scrib-
ble in my book as I tried to wrap my head around
what the doctor was saying.

It is really important to keep notes, and not just
notes from the meetings with the doctors. You will
see many doctors. You will have many tests. You will
be bombarded with information. You will have more
appointments than you can possibly comprehend.
You will become acquainted with many wonderful physician's assistants and administrative assistants and nurses and volunteers, and you will want
to remember them. You may want to write down an
observation or two about something you encounter in this strange country where you have found
yourself—Cancerland. You will have lots of phone
numbers and e-mail addresses and dates to keep
track of. I have all the latest technological gizmos,
and some were quite useful to me during my treatment. However, nothing has been as comforting as
a good old-fashioned notebook. I don't mean a jour-

nal where you pour out your most inner thoughts. I mean a notebook. A place you can just jot.

Mine was a Jane Austen notebook. In fact, I had used it to plan a trip to Bath, England, with my family, to pay homage to one of my favorite authors, so I have train times and a hotel reservation noted in it. My daughter has written down something of an itinerary—*Pump Room? Fashion Museum?*—and of course www.janeausten.co.uk. That took up just the first couple of pages. The rest was blank. So rather than buy a new book, I made this my cancer notebook. I happen to find solace in Jane Austen, so a lined notebook with pithy quotes from her was something that provided great comfort to me.

> *Friendship is certainly the finest balm for the pangs of disappointed love.*
>
> —NORTHANGER ABBEY

Well, it also happens to be the finest balm when you are going through a wretched disease, as I discovered. You should choose whatever works for you, but get something that you can easily carry with you everywhere. The thing about a notebook is that it is portable, can be beautiful, and doesn't need a Wi-Fi signal. There were moments I could have whipped out an iPad to take notes, but somehow that would have seemed a lot more obtrusive.

It is also important to realize that you will probably need a stenographer with you, particularly for the doctor appointments. As I skim through my notebook now, I see lots of my husband's spidery scrawl across the pages; clearly I was not very good at multitasking in this instance—listening and writing at the same time when my health was the topic of conversation! Almost all of the notes from doctor appointments are in my husband's hand. Phone numbers, observations, appointments are in mine. We would also write down a list of questions before an appointment so we knew exactly what to ask when we got there. Glancing back now, I see questions like *Genetic testing? Prophylactic mastectomy on the other breast?* There are the notes from various appointments like this one post-op on the final pathology report: *"found a 3rd .3cm invasive tumor . . . mastectomy was right call."* There is a double-page chart sketched out by my husband on which he tried to lay out the various possible outcomes of a test I was about to have that would determine whether or not I would have chemotherapy.

It may seem strange to say, but this notebook has become a sort of talisman for me. As I have moved further away from the original drama of diagnosis and the seemingly endless visits to the hospital for treatment, I have noticed how my notebook reflects the different stages I endured. It charts progress from diagnosis to treatment, to post-treatment. It reminds me of the people I met along the way who made things a little easier, like Mary Redding, the amazing volunteer at the chemo infusion unit, and Shawnette Morton, the gatekeeper to my plastic surgeon who managed to schedule every appointment to fit my life as well as his! As I turn the pages and see them less and less densely packed with my husband's scrawl and more and more entries in my hand, it reminds me that I have come a long way. Who knew a notebook could do that?

"O" IS FOR ODDS

If I told you that you had a one-in-eight chance of winning the lottery, you'd probably run out and buy a ticket right now. Those are extremely good odds. Odds worth acting upon for, say, betting on the Triple Crown, or the World Series or the lottery! So it is sobering to think that the odds are very good that if you are a woman in the United States of America you will get breast cancer. In fact the odds are one in eight that you will get breast cancer.

Once you are diagnosed with breast cancer, you suddenly realize that you could get really interested in statistics like that or, as my friend Linda calls it, "medical math." The two most common risk factors for breast cancer are being female and getting older. So once you are one of those one in eight, you become really interested in trying to understand odds a little better. Because actually every decision you make once you are diagnosed is predicated upon understanding the odds and acting upon that understanding. Understanding the odds of attacking the cancer if you have a lumpectomy versus a mastectomy. Understanding the odds of recurrence if you have chemotherapy followed by oral drugs after your mastectomy or if you just have the mastectomy and nothing else. Once you start the drugs *and* you start feeling the side effects, you begin thinking about what your odds would be like if you stopped taking the drugs so you could get some relief from the side effects. You are always thinking about the odds of the breast cancer coming back in five years or ten years or fifteen years. Wow, that's a lot of math to think about.

I have broken my own rule on trolling the Internet just to look at this question of odds. The National Cancer Institute has a handy little calculator called a Breast Cancer Risk Assessment Tool. According to that, my odds of getting breast cancer were 0.8 percent. Well, that didn't work out so well. I guess someone has to be in that 0.8 percent. Eighty-five percent of breast cancers occur where there is no family history—okay, I think that stat makes me feel a little better (see "G Is for Guilt").

Once I was diagnosed, what other fascinating things could I glean from statistics? There's a chart for everything. A chart for survival rates—five, ten, and fifteen years—based on the stage of your cancer.

You can look up survival rates based on age. You can examine your odds for survival depending on your race. The course of treatment to follow is also dictated by odds. A pathology of your tumor can help assess the risk of recurrence based on the treatment options *and* that pathology. What combination of treatments reduces the chance of recurrence the most? The kind of test I took, the Oncotype DX test, was supposed to help evaluate the chances of recurrence for me and my particular tumor on a spectrum of risk from low to high. The course of treatment was obvious if you were low risk or high risk. I, of course, was intermediate so had to figure out what treatment I felt I should have, since the math wasn't conclusive. I guess in that sense I'm a pretty run-of-the-mill breast cancer patient. I was never really good at this kind of math, and it can get overwhelming.

However, the dirty little secret about breast cancer is that it is all about odds. It irks me when people ask if I am "all clear" or if I am in "remission" or if I am "cured." These are words I have never heard uttered by my doctors. Not ever. Once a diagnosis is made, the doctors remove the cancer they have found, including, they hope, any microscopic cells that may be running around your body looking for another place to lodge. Then they work on trying to lower the odds of its coming back. Let's remember, there is no cure for cancer, yet. This is also why I have a problem with the word *survivor*. I have survived, for now. As the years progress, I am going to be checking the math I was so engaged in at the beginning to see how I match up. Odds that I'll be around to do *that* five years after being diagnosed? Eighty-eight percent.

"P" IS FOR
PILLOWS

Pillows are decidedly decadent. Nothing evokes sybaritic pleasures like the sight of a luxury hotel advertising its dreamy beds with a fluffy cloud of pillows. A pile of soft marshmallows that you just want to dive into and that can't possibly be good for you, can it?

Pillows date back to ancient Egypt. They've been found in tombs buried with the dead. They were decorative works of art. In ancient China they were made of hard materials like porcelain, jade, and wood, each a solid block with a half-moon cut out at the top where you could rest your neck but keep your head off the floor. Their usage has spread over the millennia, though in Tudor England they were thought to be good only for weak men and women bearing children. I've had lots of fights about pillows with my husband—how many do we really need on the bed if we can't use them all? What's a decorative pillow? Do you really need a pillow when we go camping? What's wrong with stuffing your clothes in a stuff sack and using that as a pillow?

Well, who knew that my cancer treatment would allow me to enter guilt-free pillow indulgence? In fact, therapeutic pillow indulgence was exactly what I needed and I didn't even know it.

Breast removal is a brutal assault on your body (see "M Is for Mastectomy"). I imagined it would hurt, but it *really* hurts. Try this exercise. Raise your arm to your mouth, fingers clenched like you are holding a toothbrush. That uses pectoral muscles. Hold down a loaf of bread with one hand and try to grip a knife and slice the bread with the other. Same muscles. Lie flat, then try to raise yourself without using your arms (I'm assuming you don't have abs of steel; I don't). Raise your arms and pull on a T-shirt, or take off a T-shirt for that matter. This is the moment you discover how important those muscles across your chest are, and as one of my doctors said, they "really do a number on those muscles" when they remove the breast.

In the post-surgical haze of my recovery room, the first thing I was conscious of was the fact that I felt so flattened you could probably have peeled me off the stretcher. Like something out of a Looney Tunes cartoon or the children's book character Flat Stanley, whom you could put in an envelope and mail to someone. That figure of speech "being run over by a bus" had real meaning for me now.

They did manage to peel me off the stretcher and transfer me to a hospital bed. But those beds have buttons that allow you to recline or elevate. I realized pretty quickly that I would need to be elevated all the time. Those pectoral muscles could not take lying flat. Sadly, with no such contraption at home, this angle was not going to be easy to replicate.

But lo and behold, an amazing delivery. My friend Jennifer, herself a double-mastectomy patient, delivered a giant foam wedge pillow. If you've seen fans of the Green Bay Packers with their famous Cheesehead headgear, you'll know what I mean when I say it is shaped like a giant wedge of cheese. So when we came home, I was able to lie in bed with my torso elevated at just the right angle. Really, in a million years I never would have known this. It has been a lifesaver, the anchor pillow in a group of pillows that contributed to my comfort during the worst periods after surgery and during recovery.

Another useful little pillow came courtesy of the American Cancer Society. A delivery from them included an enormous amount of literature and this three-by-six-inch pillow. What was I supposed to do with this? It might work for a big doll, but really? Well, turns out it fit pretty snugly in my armpit, where the surgeons had been ferreting around checking out my lymph nodes, and the pillow really eased the pain. The soft pillow my daughter made as part of a sewing project? Very handy to place under my side where I no longer had a breast but had plenty of pain and tenderness. Firm pillows, soft pillows, large pillows, small pillows, wedge, circle, square. The architecture of my pillow arrangement was a vital part of my treatment and recovery. I spent an inordinate amount of time in bed during my period of surgery and treatment, and I would have been lost without my pillows. In a time of enormous discomfort, pillows are an indulgence that you can afford, and they actually make a huge difference. Who knew?

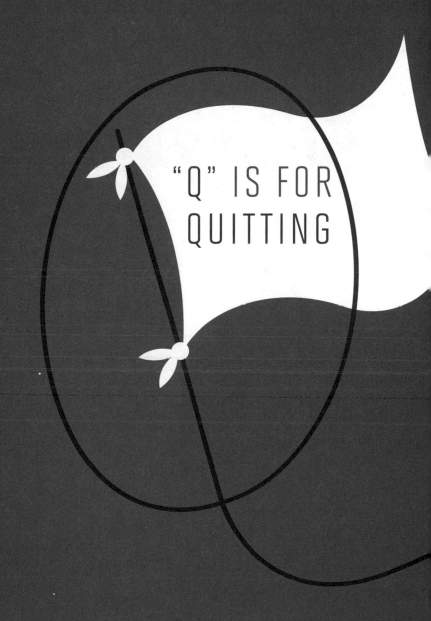

"Q" IS FOR
QUITTING

"I give up."

How many times have I said that to myself or thought that during this long, arduous thing called "breast cancer"? If I had actually tried to keep count, I'm sure I would have lost track.

Quitting comes up a lot. I don't mean in a melodramatic way of leave me alone here to die. I just mean in the getting up every day and putting one foot in front of the other as you deal with the enormity of your news and the incredible busyness of managing your disease and treatment and then actually going through the treatment. Oh, yeah, and the rest of your life continues without interruption (see "E Is for Epiphany").

In the early part of the process, the sheer number of appointments will give you pause. You need to be checked out for all your doctors—the breast surgeon, the oncologist, the plastic surgeon. It is a lot to keep track of, especially if you are one of those people who has been pretty healthy and only saw the doctor once a year.

"We need to draw blood for X."

"You need an MRI."

"We need to draw blood for Y."

"You need another biopsy, there's another mass."

"We need to draw blood for Z."

"You need to go to nuclear medicine for your MUGA scan; we want to know if your heart can stand chemo."

"Oh, yeah, we need to draw blood for X, Y, and Z."

On and on it goes, and your thoughts range from You people need to quit poking me with needles to Yes, I do mind if a medical student practices drawing blood from me.

That whole keep-moving-through-your-tiredness thing (see "X Is for eXhaustion") is another point where quitting seems to be the most attractive option.

YOU: I can't walk further than this block.

VOICE IN YOUR HEAD: You have to keep moving, just another block.

YOU: Okay, I made it to the end of this block. I need to quit now.

VOICE IN YOUR HEAD: Will yourself through the tiredness.

YOU: But doesn't turning around and walking the same distance back count?

I will confess, that whole keep-moving thing was incredibly hard for me. The days I did it I felt a tremendous sense of achievement; the days I didn't I tried to cut myself some slack.

If you lose weight during chemo, my theory is that it's not necessarily because you are throwing up. The advancement in antinausea medicine is truly extraordinary, and while I felt plenty nauseous, I didn't throw up once during chemo. I think the real culprit is your taste buds, which have been blown to smithereens by the poison. "You need to protein-load," the nutritionist told me. That's all well and good, but taste, texture, smell, everything is out of whack. I took to eating with plastic utensils because everything tasted like the metal of the silverware. The texture of yogurt *did* make me feel like I wanted to barf. Almost everything I ate left a salty taste in my mouth, including mint–chocolate chip ice cream! And the things I usually enjoyed, like the smell of broccoli stir-fried in garlic? No thank you. And the thing I love most, a nice cup of tea, was completely off the menu. I didn't drink tea during my treatment at all, and prior to that you could have described me as an addict. My day could not get going without a cup of tea. Really, why even bother? I should just quit eating and drinking.

Is there ever an acceptable moment to succumb to the desire to quit? Well, if you believe the combative rhetoric surrounding the breast cancer movement (see "W Is for Warrior"), then I guess the answer would be no. In a real-world example of cognitive dissonance, that combative rhetoric is often coupled with a gossamer pink lens through which the soldier looks at her adversary. From this vantage point, attitude is all. As if somehow your bad attitude gave you breast cancer, now a good attitude will cure it. By this logic, your attitude should be Don't quit, keep fighting, keep pushing, and you can beat this thing.

Well, sorry to be contrary, but yes, there are times when it is okay to quit. Maybe for an hour, maybe for the day. The whole doctor appointment and testing regimen thing—can't really quit that. Other things, though, hell yeah, you can give yourself permission to say no. There will be days when you will not be able to walk through that eXhaustion. That's okay. It won't be forever, and maybe taking a break will make you feel well enough to walk a bit further the next day.

Well-meaning family and friends will be plying you with "good, healthy food" that will actually make you *want* to puke. Just politely tell them you are quitting eating that for now and find what works for you and eat it to your heart's content. For me, it was peanut butter, crackers, and Gatorade. It's funny, it's a little like pregnancy; weird chemical distortions are happening to your body, and you think you will change forever. However, like pregnancy, this, too, shall pass.

And the odd day when you want to quit the world completely—no contact with anyone, getting lost in a chick flick or a book or just your own company— that is the most satisfying quitting of all.

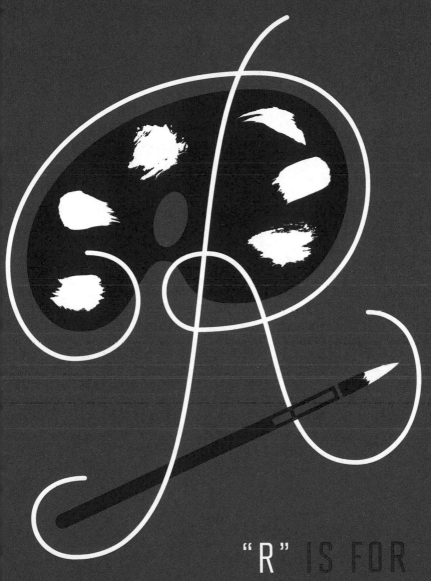

"R" IS FOR
RECONSTRUCTION

If you have had a mastectomy, the wonders of modern technology mean that you can get your breast rebuilt. It's important to remember that breast reconstruction is not the same as having a boob job. You are not someone on a bad reality TV show, looking to make up for what Mother Nature couldn't provide. This is not about vanity; it is something much more profound than that. This is an attempt to make you whole, at least cosmetically. You will actually become familiar with terms like *nip, tuck, reduce, liposuction, fat graft, implant, tattoos*—all in an effort to rebuild your breast and, indirectly, you.

My advice is to look upon your plastic surgeon as an artist who works on individual commissions, your very own Michelangelo. Every single breast he rebuilds is an original, and he will treat yours as such. Soon enough he and everyone in his office is looking at your breasts. He will ask you about size, shape, nipple, areola (that's where the tattoo comes in). He will describe how the rebuilding happens in stages.

Since it was unclear what treatment I would be going through, my doctors and I made the decision not to reconstruct at the time of the mastectomy but to get a temporary implant instead. It would be filled with saline solution, a little more each week to allow the skin to stretch to somewhere near the size of the new breast. Spoiler alert. The temporary implant feels awful. It rides high in the chest and is kind of hard. One friend described it as "like having a Fisher-Price toy stuck in your chest." That pretty much says it. The good news is it is temporary.

As you think about reconstruction, your breasts will become the center of everything, regardless of whether you gave them any thought before (see "B Is for Breasts"). They will be touched by many people in the medical profession, and you will start to touch your breasts more yourself. You will eventually look in the mirror more. Doctors will stare intently and assess your torso like a blank canvas, artists or sculptors eyeing everything before making the first stroke.

After your treatment (chemo or radiation, or both) is done, it's time to get the permanent implant, and the doctor takes to his canvas. He is creating a work of art he knows cannot be completed in one sitting. You will discuss the size of the permanent implant and how the contours of your new breast will fall. This may require several surgeries, and you prepare yourself for that. Every time he operates on you, he proceeds like a fine architect or builder. His drawings are done with the aid of nothing more complicated than a Sharpie and experience, and your chest is where he will demonstrate his skills as an artist. He will mark up what needs to happen on your chest—no measuring tapes or spirit levels, just his expert eye. And when he takes the knife to you, it should be right the first time. A few months after the implant he builds a nipple from your skin. After that he'll tattoo an areola.

He knows he cannot replicate exactly what you had, but the effort to eradicate the visual reminder of what has happened to you is quite extraordinary. You have lost your breast, of course. There is no feeling. There will be no feeding. Other doctors will marvel at the good work he has performed—clean incisions, tight stitching, fast healing. Every day you look in the mirror, as the scarring begins to fade, it is not a deformity that faces you but a remarkable work of art.

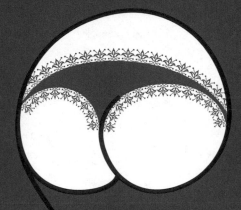

"S" IS FOR SEX

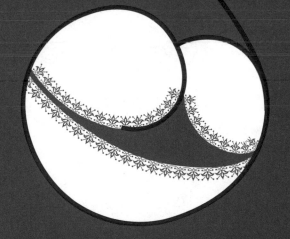

Cancerland is a place where, as the late Christopher Hitchens put it, "there seems to be almost no talk of sex." In the case of breast cancer, he was right. Now I don't want to get all cancer competitive on you, but the discussion of prostate cancer is often accompanied by concerns about its impact on a man's sex life. With breast cancer, if there is any discussion of sex at all, it is likely to be if you are of childbearing age, and it is more likely to be about *fertility* than it is about *sexuality*. Your sex life doesn't come up much.

If this is not an issue for you, I applaud you and recommend you move on to "T Is for Therapy."

If this is an issue for you, let's talk about it. As you've gleaned from the preceding pages, when the complete embodiment of your womanhood—your breasts—becomes diseased, this is not an easy thing to deal with. In fact, sex is so far from your mind that you might be asking yourself, Why is she bringing this up at all? The National Cancer Institute reports, "About half of women who have long-term treatment for breast and reproductive organ cancers . . . report long-term sexual problems." So if you are going through any sexual challenges during treatment, you are in good company. But every year, hundreds of thousands of women are treated for breast cancer and come out the other side. While sex may be on hiatus during treatment, it doesn't have to stop forever.

Lots of things can affect your sex drive when you are diagnosed with breast cancer. First, you've been diagnosed with breast cancer (see "A Is for Anxiety")! There is nothing that can prepare you for the number that does on you mentally. This is news that you need time to cope with, and really, all your attention can be focused on that for as long as you need.

Second, if you have breast surgery, you hurt. You hurt physically because some or all of your breast or breasts have been removed. That is a whole lot of hurt (see "M Is for Mastectomy"), not to mention bandages and drains and general yuckiness. I've tried to think of any way to interpret this immediate post-surgical period as sexy, but I really can't. Please let me know if I am wrong. You hurt emotionally too. Not only are you in mourning for the previously healthy you, but you are in mourning for a part of your body that may have helped define your sexiness, appeal, attractiveness. It is really hard to get aroused when you are in that kind of state.

Third, you might have to undergo chemotherapy and/or radiation. How do I begin to describe the un-sexiness of that? Your body is being pumped with toxic chemicals and countless other drugs to counter the effects of the toxic chemicals. Here are some of the side effects that were possible from the particu-lar chemo that I was taking:

- Fluid retention with weight gain, swelling of the ankles or abdominal area
- Peripheral neuropathy (numbness in your fingers and toes)
- Nausea
- Diarrhea
- Mouth sores
- Hair loss
- Fatigue and weakness
- Infection
- Nail changes, including in extreme cases nails falling off

Nothing sexy about any of that list!

So you go through the weeks and months of surgery and recovery, followed by chemotherapy and recovery, maybe followed by radiation and recovery. During that time you will want to be loved and hugged and calmed and comforted, and maybe you will want to have sex. But maybe you won't. This is where the U Is for Understanding (see "U Is for Un-") comes in on the part of your partner. Your partner may not feel that you are deformed or unsexy or unattractive. In fact your partner may be working hard to convince you of the exact opposite, that you are as beautiful and lovely as you were when love first struck, that a surgery like this, and the resultant nine-inch scar across your chest, and your baldness and your bloating, changes none of that. Your partner means it. You just might not be in a condition to hear any of it.

One of my doctors did bring it up with me actually.

DOCTOR: How is your sex life?
ME: Um, nonexistent.

DOCTOR: I know it's hard but . . .

ME: It's *really* hard, I feel like crap.

DOCTOR: I know, but it's like a muscle, you have to keep using it!

There you have it, the view from a medical professional. So while not many people talk about it, a lot of the cancer literature will deal with the question of *intimacy*. It's important enough that the National Cancer Institute lists intimacy as one of the parts of your life that can be severely affected by a diagnosis of cancer. And that is the first step, recognizing that your sex life, sort of like your taste buds and your energy level and your hair, is affected by your treatment. Like all of those things, it comes back. It just comes back on its own timetable. And I speak from experience.

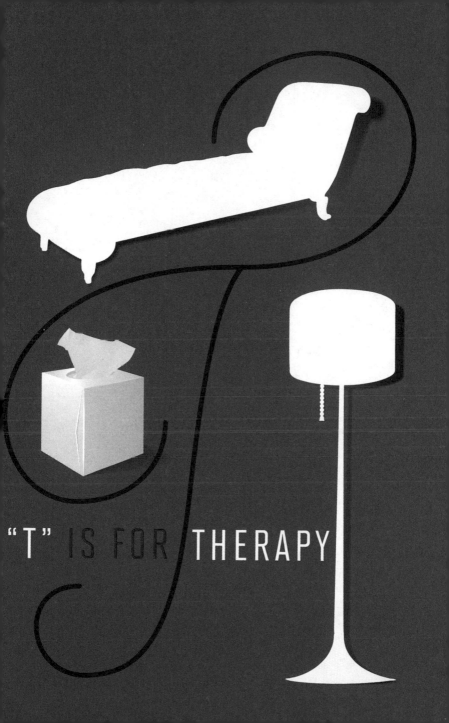

"T" IS FOR THERAPY

My love affair with *Downton Abbey* began when I was diagnosed with breast cancer. It was during that interminable period after your biopsy confirms what you feared but before you know exactly what the doctors want to do about it. It was also that interminable period between Christmas and New Year's. Almost everyone is away and you are awaiting the results of more pathologies from more tests and all you are able to do is hurry up and wait.

My friends at PBS had sent me an advance screener of this new British costume drama, which was to premiere in the new year. I have a soft spot for such things, and since I didn't have much to do but fret about the what-ifs, I threw the disc into my computer and started to watch. Resting comfortably on my bed, my laptop perched on a breakfast tray, I proceeded to indulge in what is now commonly called "binge viewing." One episode after another, I got lost in the scandalous saga of Lady Mary and Mr. Pamuk and Lady Sybil's idealism and Mr. Bates's repression and Lord Grantham's propriety. There were dark clouds on the horizon (for the inhabitants of *Downton Abbey* as well as for me), but for now we could be consumed by trifles that took on such profound meaning. No doctor could have ordered this escapism for me. It was probably the best therapy I could have had at that particular moment. And yes, I watched it twice!

My point is, when you are diagnosed with breast cancer, you face months of therapy, maybe years. But here's the thing: there are all sorts of therapies, and my advice would be to avail yourself of them *all* and whenever necessary.

There is, of course, the biggie—chemotherapy. Generally you don't get a choice in the matter; your genes are calling the shots here. If you have a mastectomy or any other kind of surgery related to your breast cancer, then physical therapy is in your future. I guess you could choose to forgo this particular therapy, but that's probably not wise (though your insurance company may make this a challenge). There's also the other drug therapy *after* the chemotherapy, you know, the one that is supposed to stop the cancer from coming back. These are all the therapies where your doctor is in the driver's seat.

And here's another one that is on your doctor's

dance card—psychotherapy. That's one that doesn't get a lot of attention in the gauzy breast cancer world of pink ribbons and sexy, glamorous cancer warriors fighting back. You will tire of the bromides about your being able to kick the ass of this disease and vanquish it, or whatever other martial language people want to use (see "W Is for Warrior"). Well, breast cancer is a bitch. Being able to say that out loud to someone, someone who will help you cope and even help you mourn, is a huge help (see "A Is for Anxiety"). So psychotherapy is nothing to be ashamed of or reluctant to embrace. It is all part of the healing. You were diagnosed with an insidious disease, your body has been maimed and poisoned and your hair has fallen out, and you feel like crap. Really, it's a wonder you didn't think about talking through all that right from the get-go.

So what else works for you? Retail therapy perhaps? Yes, this is one of those therapies for which women get a bad rap. Well, I have some good news: this is the kind of therapy you never have to feel guilty about when you have breast cancer (see "F Is for Fashion Accessories"). I can vouch for the therapeutic benefits of shopping for particular items that will make you feel better about yourself. Honest. Along with my pillow therapy (see "P Is for Pillows"), we bought a new mattress. That's one of those things we'd thought about for ages. Now I knew I was going to spend a lot of time in bed recuperating and resting, why shouldn't I have a comfortable mattress? Indulgent? Maybe. Therapeutic? Absolutely.

I will admit that there have been times in my life when I have found eating to be therapeutic. This one is a little tougher when you are undergoing chemotherapy. Your taste buds have undergone a strange chemical metamorphosis that plays havoc with flavor and texture and smell. But when the moment strikes you and you must eat (fill in the blank), have at it. My nutritionist wanted me to eat whatever I wanted and whatever stayed down. For the first time in my life, guilt-free ice cream! Just what the doctor ordered.

Here are some other things that were incredibly therapeutic for me: flowers, friends, serialized television dramas like *Downton Abbey* and *John Adams* (because I had no energy to watch a whole movie in one sitting—I had to watch *Eat, Pray, Love* in three sittings and wish I had stopped after *Eat*), every single member of my family who came to visit, especially my toddler nephew, my work (when I was up for it), reading when I could, and crying, seemingly at random.

Therapy is all about healing, and the beauty of healing is that it can apply to your body, your soul, your mind, and your surroundings. And finding therapy the doctor doesn't have to prescribe and insurance doesn't have to pay for is probably the best of all.

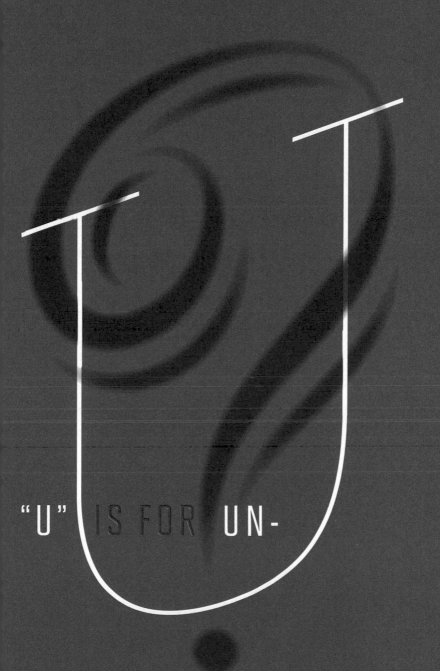

"U" IS FOR UN-

Yes, I know, this is a prefix. But here's the thing: I couldn't decide on which *un-* since there are so many! The first one is *understanding*. There are so many things you need to understand when you have breast cancer. You need to *understand* that it is *unfair* and it is *uncertain* and it is *unpredictable* and it seems *unending*.

It is *unfair*. On hearing your diagnosis, this will probably be one of your first thoughts. You will not think about that list of possible factors for breast cancer (see "G Is for Guilt"), you will just think about the cruel hand of fate that has dealt you this blow. The reality is, it *is* unfair that you have breast cancer. There is no logic to it. In the majority of cases there isn't even a genetic explanation for it. It just is (see "O Is for Odds"). The cosmic answer to "why me?" is "why not?"

Uncertainty will pursue you in Cancerland, nipping at your heels like an irritating, yapping little dog that you actually want to kick away but can't. Should I get a second opinion? Should I shave off my hair? Should I have a prophylactic mastectomy? Should I have the most aggressive treatment even if the pathologies are inconclusive? At some point you will be uncertain about every single decision that you make.

How you are going to react to your treatment is somewhat *unpredictable,* at least to begin with. If you are having surgery, it might take you longer to bounce back than your doctor tells you. Everyone's reaction to chemotherapy is different too. Your doctor can list all the possible side effects that come from the chemo, and she may even sound like one of those disclaimers they throw on the ends of commercials for drugs while she does it. Yet it is hard to predict which ones will hit you. If you *understand* this seeming *unpredictability,* you might find some patterns. After your first chemo session, keep notes on how you react and when. You're likely to see a pattern as you progress through the sessions, and *understanding* that goes halfway to helping you deal with it.

Every single thing about going through breast cancer will, at some point, strike you as *unending.* And indeed, when you are going through all this crap, it is *unending.* As I've mentioned before in this book, the constant round of medical appointments seems *unending,* and that's before you've even started your treatment. Once you've gone through surgery and chemo, you might face weeks of daily radiation—*that* can seem *unending.* And then when you've gone through all your treatment, the *uncertainty* of whether the cancer will come back again is *unending* and thus something you have to manage. All I can tell you is that you will get to the other side. It may not seem like it when you are in the thick of it, but it is true. Some of this crap really does come to an end.

So, what you need most in your life, at this time, is some *understanding* in all its meaning. Obviously you need to understand what is happening to you, the status of your disease, and the plan to treat it. You can also look for some *understanding* from those around you as you go through your treatment. Help them understand what you are going through and what you are feeling. This is the only way for everyone to get through it.

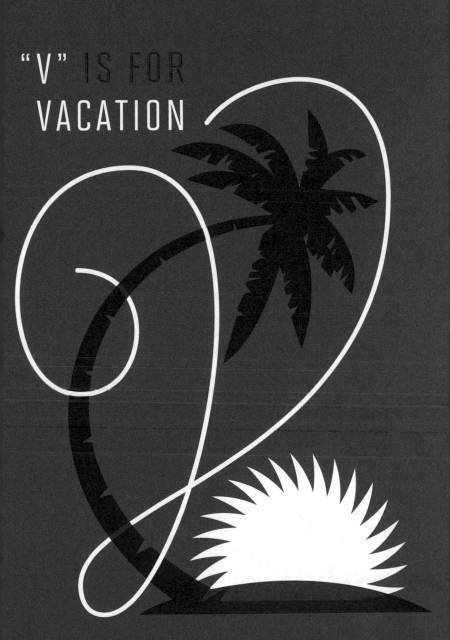

"V" IS FOR
VACATION

Yes, I know vacation is the farthest thing from your mind. You are already visiting this strange new place called Cancerland, a foreign destination hard to navigate, a place you are never really going to leave. How could you possibly be thinking about a vacation? Well, I consider a vacation an admirable goal to strive for during the worst of your treatment. I did, and it was worth it.

When you are diagnosed with breast cancer, your doctors and larger medical team—there are so many of them—will become among the most important people in your life. There are so many appointments to keep; so many tests to undergo; so much pain, nausea, and discomfort to endure. I certainly felt that I wanted to be close to my doctors at all times, day or night. The anxiety of the what-ifs is palpable. When you are undergoing treatment you are, well, sick. Sometimes you might get so sick that you need to go to the hospital. I ended up in the emergency room twice while I was undergoing chemotherapy, glad that the hospital was just a short ride away.

There are ups during each cycle of chemotherapy, when you tell yourself you are feeling better and you can do anything. But then you remember that your immune system is completely and utterly compromised. I once entertained the thought of attending an event in New York during one of these upswings. I was sure I had the energy and thought that taking the train from Washington, D.C., to New York would be less taxing than flying. Then I started to think about the circle of germs I would encounter on that trip—touching door handles, breathing in the same air as a train car full of people, arriving at Penn Station and encountering the full panoply of what New York City has to offer at that particular crossroads of humanity. (For the uninitiated, it is not the most welcoming of major city train stations; in fact, it is old, and murky, and dirty, and thoroughly depressing.) Since I couldn't guarantee a Purell perimeter zone with me in it and everyone else out of it, staying close to home seemed to make most sense for me.

So, would I ever get beyond a three-mile radius of my house? Well, it turned out that eventually I would. What I needed was a goal. For years I had wanted to visit Istanbul. In fact, one of my earliest thoughts upon diagnosis was I'm going to die and I've never been to Istanbul. So for me, finally taking that vacation was a worthy thing to strive for. During the real lows of my treatment, it seemed the most unattainable thing possible but also, on some days, the only thing I might get out of bed for. Ah, the paradox of cancer treatment.

But your vacation doesn't have to be in a destination as exotic as that. A change of scenery is a great thing, even for a day or two, but it *must* be a vacation for you. I made the mistake of making a work trip out of town too soon and ran myself ragged and had to come home early. A few months after chemotherapy the first pleasure trip I took was to visit friends in Massachusetts. Here are the things I remember about that trip: I was leaving home, so I was leaving my cancer behind for a while; they were really good friends and there were no expectations on either side, they just wanted me to get away for a break and I wanted to be somewhere different; I was really tired; I spent a lot of the weekend on the couch in their living room, the sea visible through the screen doors, and I let the salty breeze drift over me; I let my friends look after me (see "K Is for Kindness"). It was forty-eight hours of bliss (see "T Is for Therapy").

There has been much talk of America's inability to take a vacation. We take less time off than any other developed nation. And we are continuously "connected" when we are vacationing, so are we really vacationing anyway? When you are undergoing cancer treatment, the restorative and rejuvenating powers of a vacation suddenly begin to make real sense. Whether for a few hours, a few days, or a few weeks, when your mind and body are ready to take that vacation—take it.

I did get to Istanbul eventually. It was everything I'd hoped it would be and more. It was my vacation from Cancerland.

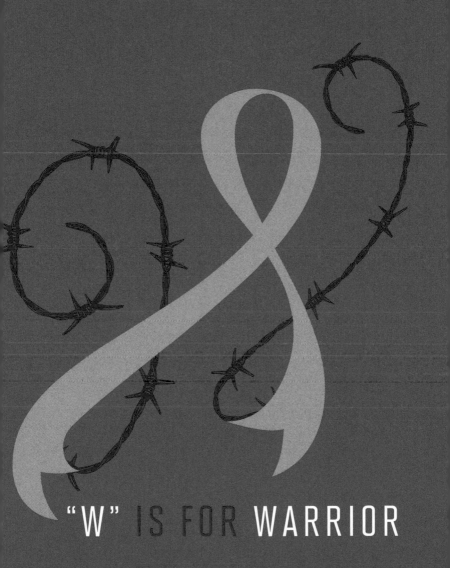

"W" IS FOR WARRIOR

I am not a warrior.

I am a journalist—my profession.

I am a wife—my status.

I am a mother—my devotion.

I am not a warrior.

However, as a breast cancer patient I am deemed to be a warrior in an army made up entirely of conscripts. I have been pressed into battle, part of the "war against cancer." We patients are the frontline infantry in this fight. We (breast cancer patients) have benefited enormously from the extraordinary effort made by millions to put breast cancer on the map. Our insignia is the pink ribbon, and we must wear it proudly. The language evoked is inevitably military. I will battle this disease. I will defeat it. I will kick the enemy's ass. But even conscripts in a regular army get some training. We, on the other hand, start our fight the second we are diagnosed. No training sessions, no time for mental preparation. I am a warrior now, a reluctant one, but desertion is not an option. I am now engaged in a war. Who is going to help me with the battle plan? How will I strategize my victory? Who is going to finance this war? Who is going to be my logistics team? I must gird myself for the fight.

But I am not a woman warrior. I am just a woman, a woman who has been diagnosed with a horrible disease; a woman who has gone through brutal surgery; a woman who has had her body poisoned to "kill" the disease. Can I just be a woman who is going through that? Can I not be a woman warrior? Please?

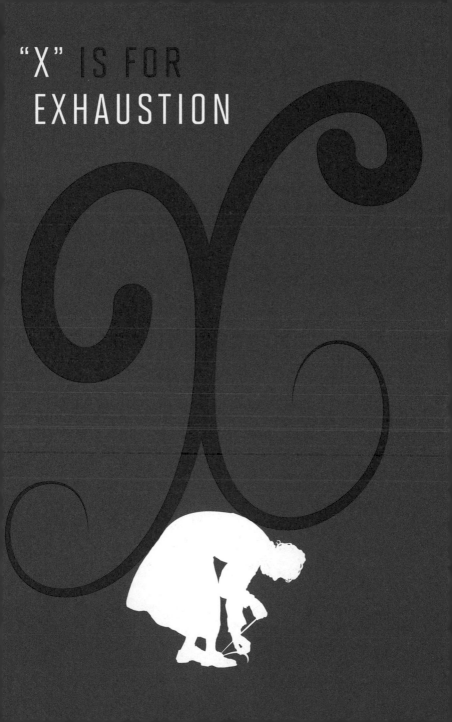

"X" IS FOR
EXHAUSTION

We have all been tired in our lives. I have given birth to two children. I have traveled the globe to cover stories where you land and start working immediately, time zone be damned. I have worked without pause, forty-eight hours, seventy-two hours in a row, just going as the adrenaline somehow keeps me pumped, and I will not be defeated by my body's greedy thirst for rest. I have gone on hikes with my husband that I have not wanted to do, when I feel that one foot will not reach in front of the other and I will be stuck on a mountaintop until an air rescue mission arrives. I am tired. Leave me alone.

When you undergo chemotherapy, the doctors will tell you about the fatigue. Or as my oncologist put it, "You won't be living that Washington professional working mother life for a while; something has to give." She means you will be exhausted. Not fatigued like a delicate Victorian damsel. You will be exhausted in a way that you cannot think is humanly possible. It is a strange kind of tiredness. At times your body cannot hold itself up. You are a rag doll. Your brain says yes but your body flops rather than flipping to attention. The poisons are coursing through your system; that wretched chemotherapy makes itself felt in every part of your body. You can't grip because your fingertips tingle from the drugs; your toes tingle too. Your joints have no adhesion. Does my knee really join my calf to my thigh? I can't tell. I want to knit but my wrists and elbows have their own ideas. Throughout it all my brain is completely and utterly awake. I have to take "rests" in the afternoon because my body won't keep up with the inside of my head. My thumbs can occasionally work on the BlackBerry; my fingers can sometimes dial a phone.

I want to fight through the exhaustion. In those early weeks of the chemotherapy, I would take a walk around the block, propped up by my husband or one of my daughters. It is one of the most counterintuitive things—walk through the exhaustion, just to keep the circulation going. I was diligent about this, but it didn't stop the exhaustion; I guess it just kept some tone in my body. It is an accomplishment to sit downstairs at the table for dinner. As the body acclimates to the treatment, the fatigue takes hold. Day 4 or 5 after a day of chemo infusion was the worst for me. The chemo, the post-chemo drugs to build up your white blood cell count to stave off infection, the fact that eating does not feel good or taste good— all these things conspire to drag you down, and this time your exhaustion feels legitimate.

You are not being a wuss. You are undergoing a radical chemical assault on your body. You have to ac- knowledge the exhaustion and just go with it. There will be days when you feel great. On the days you don't, just let it be. It is not about you, it is about the chemicals. Of course, the more chemo you have, the worse it gets. The effects are cumulative. And what you are not quite prepared for is that it stays with you well after your last chemo session. How long? Six months? A year? Two? It is different for everyone. Your exhaustion is not a reflection of you or of any weakness on your part. It is a testament to the power of the drugs that are out there chasing every one of those bad cells away. Unfortunately, they chase the good cells too. Cut yourself some slack and take as much rest as you need. You deserve it.

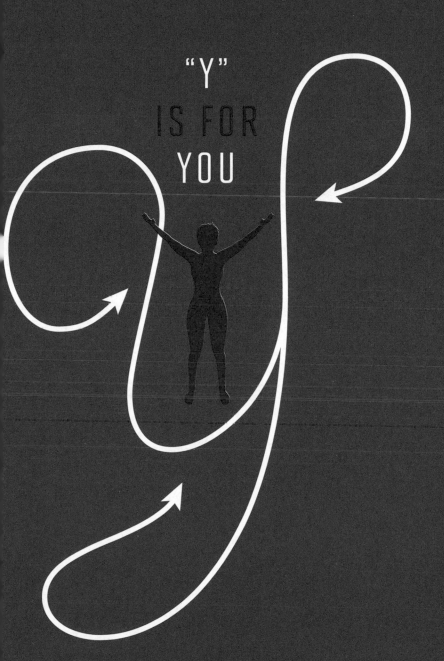

I don't think I am a particularly selfish person. I have a husband and two children, so I consider three other people in my life every single day. Growing up in a house with three siblings meant that even on the days when I might have wanted things to be about me, they weren't. I work in a business where absolutely nothing gets done without the collaboration of so many others. This has made me conscious of people around me and able to interact in myriad situations with myriad individuals.

When you are diagnosed with breast cancer, however, it is all about *you*. This is the most rare of situations when you have permission to be selfish and self-centered and maybe even a bit demanding. This doesn't mean you should turn into a bitch. It means you should surrender to the fact that you have this terrible diagnosis and you really need to focus on you and what you need. What you are feeling at any given moment is the most important thing during this period. Give yourself permission to get comfortable with that.

A focus on you can take many forms. For your family, your disease and treatment become the "thing," the dominant force in your family's life. For our family this meant a calendar chockablock with appointments and tests for me, many of which my husband had to be a part of, sometimes because I needed someone to bring me home, sometimes to be the second set of ears, listening in on every conversation with every medical professional (see "N Is for Notebook"). So his focus had to be on me. It meant my siblings and my sister-in-law and my father all came from overseas just for me. Not as they had so many times before, to see my growing children, or to take a vacation from work and see the cherry blossoms in D.C., but to see me and help me with whatever I needed.

There were more mundane ways in which my focus on myself was felt by all. Beware my wrath if you finished up the only ice cream flavor that I could eat. Okay, maybe I was a bitch about that. If I didn't want to have people drop by, I could just say no without a sense of guilt or obligation or impropriety or anything else. If I wanted to spend the afternoon in bed crying, well, that was okay too.

My recommendation to you is to embrace *you,*

which is harder than it sounds. At many points in your life, perhaps in a moment of quiet reflection, you might have admitted to yourself that what you wanted to say was "to heck" with everyone else, here is what I want to do. Breast cancer gives you the perfect excuse to do this, although going through with it will make you feel terrible. Terrible because you feel that this disease is now a burden to so many other people and you feel guilty about it (see "G Is for Guilt"). You might feel a little timid about being demanding. Don't. It is perfectly appropriate to have your world turn its direction toward you. It is a useful advantage of carrying the cancer card—use it to its utmost benefit.

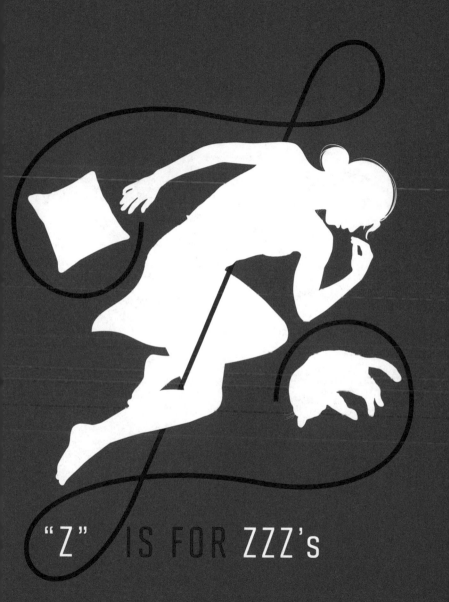

"Z" IS FOR ZZZ's

Catching some zzz's is a cartoonish way of describing sleep. In fact, it was the only way for a cartoonist to connote sleep (and not death) almost a century ago. Capital ZZZ's, maybe punctuated by an exclamation point, were supposed to replicate the gentle sound of snoring. So simple and so effective when you see them in a cartoon panel.

Sadly, there is nothing comical or simple about your relationship with sleep when you become a cancer patient. In fact, it seems as if there is a vast conspiracy allied against you and your ability to sleep. Your mom always told you that you needed a "good night's sleep," and there's plenty of research to support the idea that sleep is one of the most restorative things you can do to maintain a healthy body and mind. And admit it, sleep is probably something you have always aspired to in the hurly-burly of your daily demands.

Ah, to sleep, perchance to dream? Actually, I'd take sleep without any dreaming. Sleep deprivation seems to be the affliction of modern America, and it is even more common when you enter Cancerland. The cabal lined up against your sleep is pretty formidable, thwarting every effort you may have in mind. You enter a vicious cycle of sleep you can't get to heal and then your inability to sleep compounds itself, and the cycle continues.

So who exactly are these conspirators stymieing your best efforts? A veritable alphabet soup of challengers, many of which you have met in the pages of this book.

There is A for Anxiety, your companion from the first moment you feel a lump or learn about an irregular mammogram; C for Cancerland—a place you never, ever wanted to visit, but now that you are there it keeps you up at night; D for the Drugs—you are taking so many of them, and some make you tired, some make you nauseous, some make you buzzed, and some you hope are killing the cancer; G for the Guilt you are feeling about so many things, like What did I do wrong to deserve this?; I for Indignities, of which there are so many once you start on this breast cancer odyssey; M for Mastectomy—it hurts so much that it defeats sleep at every turn, including, literally, if you want to sleep on your stomach; R for Reconstruction—so many surgeries, messing up every natural rhythm that your body ever possessed; S for the Sex you feel bad about not having because you feel like crap and hurt like hell; X for the eXhaustion you are feeling throughout this whole ordeal but are too exhausted to sleep.

And of course sometimes these conspirators form a tight-knit brigade, like Anxiety fed by Guilt, which is exacerbated by not wanting Sex. You get the picture: so many forces marshaled against your ability to sleep.

So where are the opposing forces, ready to do battle against the formidable enemies of sleep? Well, you've met some of them in the pages of this book too. D, that traitor, can be found on both sides of the battlefield, because you can get Drugs to help you sleep. Don't worry about becoming addicted, get some sleep; they may not always work perfectly, but they're a start. P for the Pillows that can make you a little more comfortable while M for Mastectomy is doing its darnedest to thwart you and your efforts to sleep at every turn. K will help you sleep too—the Kindness of others will soothe the darkest moments that are feeding your anxiety; thinking about V for

Vacation can take you out of the Cancerland you are visiting now to a place where you really want to be that will replenish and rejuvenate you.

It is important to remember there will be replenishment and rejuvenation. But it will not happen fast, and it will not happen the way you think it might. Dealing with breast cancer happens not on your timetable but on the timetable of the disease. What you *do* have control of is how you deal with it and how you want to cope. And getting some shut-eye, however you can, is one of the best ways of all to cope.

POSTSCRIPT

It is possible that there is no more beautiful place in Washington during the Christmas holidays than the White House. Each year the president and first lady open up the mansion to thousands of visitors, including the press, to celebrate the season. In a rather extraordinary twist of fate, exactly one year to the day after learning about my cancer while standing on the driveway outside the press briefing room, I returned to the White House to attend one of those parties. Since that chilly evening a year earlier, I had undergone a mastectomy, the awfulness of chemotherapy, reconstructive surgery with more to come, drugs as a daily part of my life, not to mention the sometimes demoralizing adjustment to my looks. In my darkest moments I hadn't looked too far ahead, certainly not to a year later and a return to the White House.

Despite the fact that I was to undergo another surgery in a week, it was a delight to revel in the joys of the season. The decorations in the White House are a sight to behold, bright and bold, meaningful and merry. From the tree honoring military personnel in the Blue Room to the cameos by the first dog, Bo, in every room in the house (including a Bo made of buttons and a Bo made of garbage bags), everything was lovely. I tried to remember everything I saw because the last time I'd been in the White House was such a blur. But the thing I remembered most was that I was standing here, with a good prognosis in front of me and blessed to have endured the previous year.

It is a strange thing about cancer: even after all your treatment it never quite leaves you, at least in the metaphorical sense. I see doctors regularly. I take drugs daily and will continue to do so for the next few years. And always in the back of my mind there's the nagging question: Will it come back? That, of course, is unknowable. But having endured once, I'll know a little of what to expect. For those of you who are enduring now, I hope that this book will have provided some comfort and solace. Everyone's cancer is unique, but my hope is that this book has provided a little something for each of you.

ACKNOWLEDGMENTS

A diagnosis of breast cancer is a diagnosis no woman wants to hear. However, if she must hear it, then I hope she will be as fortunate as I have been in the medical professionals who have been with me throughout. They are Dr. Rebecca Evangelista, Dr. Claudine Isaacs, Dr. Maurice Nahabedian, Dr. Lauren Randel. A very special thank-you to my general internist, Dr. Margot Wheeler. If everybody in America were as fortunate in their internists, then we could all feel a little better about our health-care system. It is not, of course, only the doctors who are your staunchest companions in this ordeal. I will be forever grateful for the kindness and grace of my oncology nurse, Sue Bergfalk, and oncology infusion unit volunteer Mary Redding. I've decided that physicians are sometimes only as good as their assistants, and so a heartfelt shout-out to Physician's Assistants Megan Fay and Kara Lee. And to all the administrators who help make smooth the path of cancer treatment, thank you, most especially Sheila Coker and Shawnette Morton.

The decision to work while undergoing cancer treatment may seem stoic to some and foolhardy to others. However, as with so much else in life, it is not possible to do without the support of many. In my case thanks are due to the past and present boss ladies of NPR, Vivian Schiller, Debra Delman, Ellen McDonnell, and Margaret Low Smith. The amazing staff of *Morning Edition* proved to me that the bonds of the workplace can endure whatever the challenges, and this is especially true for my extraordinary management team: Tracy Wahl, Cara Tallo, Shannon Rhoades, Kitty Eisele, and Chuck Holmes. I am forever in their debt.

I am grateful to the fellow cancer sufferers who shared their triumphs and tribulations with me and helped me face my darkest fears—Meri Kolbrener, Jennifer Griffin, and Eileen Murphy.

There is something about the bonds of friendship that becomes tighter in the face of challenge and hardship, and that is true of my ladies of the book club. Kathryn Kross, Jill Rosenbaum, Sara Just, and Su-Lin Nichols, thank you.

To my family who crossed the pond in turns, so

someone was always here. Dad, sorry to put you through this hellish ordeal, but the good news is I must have got my toughness from someone. Meera, Sujata, and Kanjeev—of the many things we've had to deal with as siblings, I know this one was the furthest from our minds, but as with everything else in our lives, you were my strength and succor.

The path from being diagnosed with breast cancer to writing a book about breast cancer is not a straight one, nor is it one to embark upon without the support of numerous people who believe in you and the story you have to tell.

Michele Norris, my friend and my sister away from my sisters, nudged this project from the first, with the presentation of blank notebooks large and small to encourage me to write. It is fair to say that without her this book would have remained a flight of fancy in my head. My friend and colleague Steve Inskeep has always believed in me and my abilities, and author was just one more title he thought I could wear. They both were my cheerleaders and helped me over the finish line.

The refuge provided by Joan Reeves, Caroline

Reeves, and Jim Lee helped me write, literally. I thank them for providing me space both physical and mental.

My darling friend David Rakoff, a seasoned cancer patient himself at the time of my diagnosis, provided all sorts of wisdom and wisecracks from day one. His thoughtfulness, even while undergoing his own extensive treatment, knew no bounds. A call the night before a major surgery or test, an e-mail to check in, a dietary tip or two, David was the best cancer friend a girl could have. He was also one of the best friends one could have in life, and I am profoundly saddened that cancer took him from us before he could see this book, which he did so much to support and nurture.

My agents, Howard Yoon and Gail Ross, always believed, of course, and this book would not be real without them. The wonderful people at Crown Publishing—Maya Mavjee, Molly Stern, and David Drake—have been my champions from the moment they saw the proposal.

In addition, many others at Crown have nurtured and shepherded the publication of this book: Jay

Sones, Jessica Prudhomme, Annsley Rosner, Claire Potter, Miriam Chotiner-Gardner, Wade Lucas, and the wonderful Rachel Rokicki. The fact that this is more than a book but a beautiful object is thanks to designers Chris Brand and Elizabeth Rendfleisch at Crown. The extraordinary illlustrations by Roberto de Vicq de Cumpitch speak to my words in a way I could never have imagined.

A relationship with an editor can be fraught with difficulty or it can foster trust. Fortunately, the literary gods teamed me up with Vanessa Mobley, an editor who was my partner, helping steer me on the path of book writing without yanking the wheel out of my hands and taking over. Vanessa, I have benefited from your guidance.

The people who have lived my cancer every day are, of course, my daughters and my husband. Living with a news mom and news wife in the house all these years required a particular forbearance, but a cancer mom and cancer wife was a whole new challenge. Priya and Maya, you were young girls when this diagnosis befell us, and your initial fear gave way to a steeliness that I think you still don't know you possessed. How proud I am of you both, particularly your strength in not being freaked out by your bald mom, a possible trauma for many a teen or pre-teen girl!

Jim, in more than a quarter century of marriage we have endured an awful lot, and have tested the vow of "in sickness and in health" to its limit. For being my stenographer and nursemaid and editor and companion and worrier, and most important, for being the love of my life, thank you.

BIBLIOGRAPHY

Alford, Henry. "Laughing at the Big C." *New York Times,* October 7, 2011.

Blume, Lesley M. M. *Let's Bring Back: An Encyclopedia of Forgotten-Yet-Delightful Chic, Useful, Curious, and Otherwise Commendable Things from Times Gone By.* Chronicle Books, 2010.

Ehrenreich, Barbara. "Welcome to Cancerland." *Harper's,* November 2001.

Hitchens, Christopher. *Mortality.* Twelve, 2012.

Leopold, Ellen. *A Darker Ribbon: Breast Cancer, Women, and Their Doctors in the Twentieth Century.* Beacon Press, 1999.

Mukherjee, Siddhartha. *The Emperor of All Maladies: A Biography of Cancer.* Scribner, 2010.

National Cancer Institute. "Breast Cancer Risk Assessment Tool." http://www.cancer.gov/bcrisktool/.

——. *Facing Forward: Life After Cancer Treatment.* NIH Publication No. 10-2424, 2010.

Olson, James S. *Bathsheba's Breast: Women, Cancer, and History.* Johns Hopkins University Press, 2002.

An indispensable and approachable guide to life during, and after, breast cancer

The biggest risk factor for breast cancer is simply being a woman. Madhulika Sikka's *A Breast Cancer Alphabet* offers a new way to live with and plan past the hardest diagnosis that most women will ever receive: a personal, practical, and deeply informative aid to coping, from diagnosis to treatment and beyond.

What Madhulika Sikka didn't foresee when initially diagnosed, and what this book brings to life so vividly, are the unexpected and minute challenges that make navigating the world of breast cancer all the trickier. *A Breast Cancer Alphabet* is an inspired reaction to what started as a personal predicament.

This A-to-Z guide to living with breast cancer goes where so many fear to tread: sex (S is for Sex—really?), sentimentality (J is for Journey—it's a cliché we need to dispense with), hair (H is for Hair—yes, you can make a federal case of it), and work (Q is for Quitting—there'll be days when you feel like it). She draws an easy-to-follow, and quite memorable, map of her travels from breast cancer neophyte to seasoned veteran.

As a prominent news executive, Madhulika had access to the most cutting-edge data on the disease's reach and impact. At the same time, she craved the community of frank talk and personal insight that we rely on in life's toughest moments. This wonderfully inventive book navigates the world of science and story, bringing readers into Madhulika's mind and experience in a way that demystifies breast cancer and offers new hope for those living with it.